Mind · Body · Bowl

Annie Clarke

Thorsons

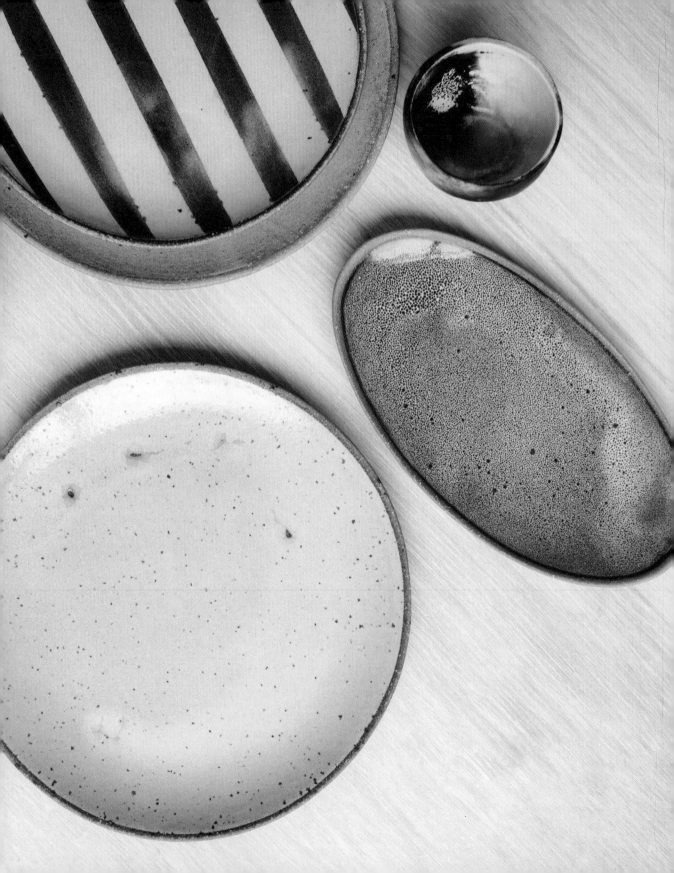

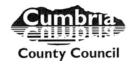
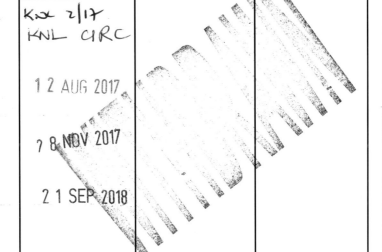

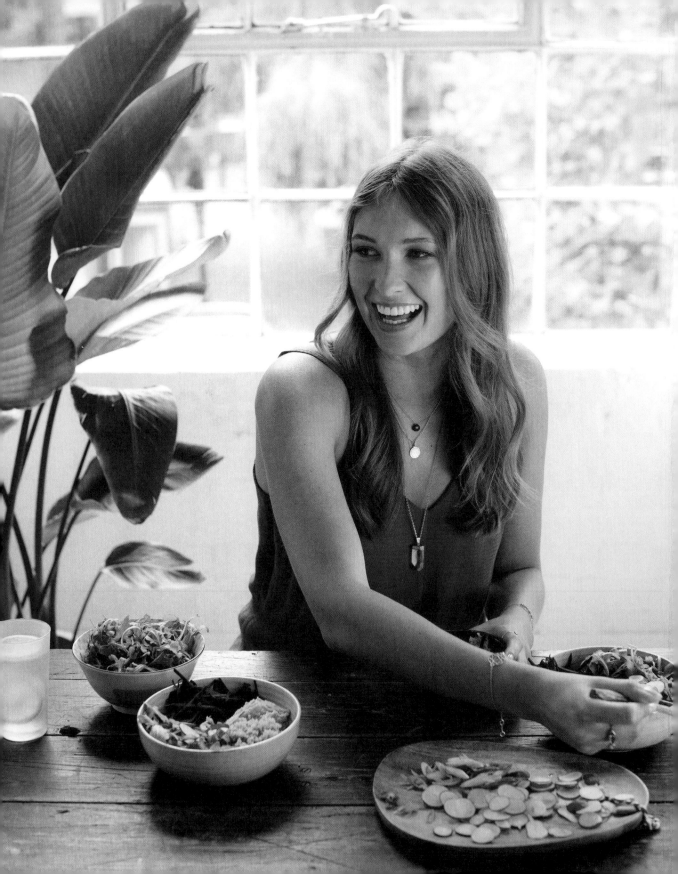

Contents

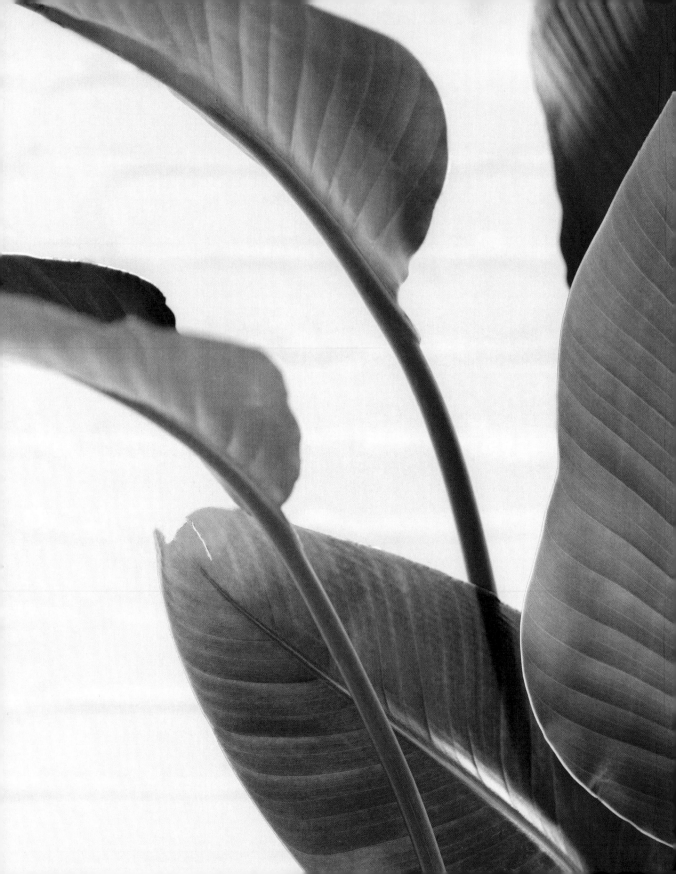

Introduction

The world of health and well-being
is growing rapidly, and it is such
an exciting time as more and more
people take a positive interest in
leading healthier, more fulfilled lives.

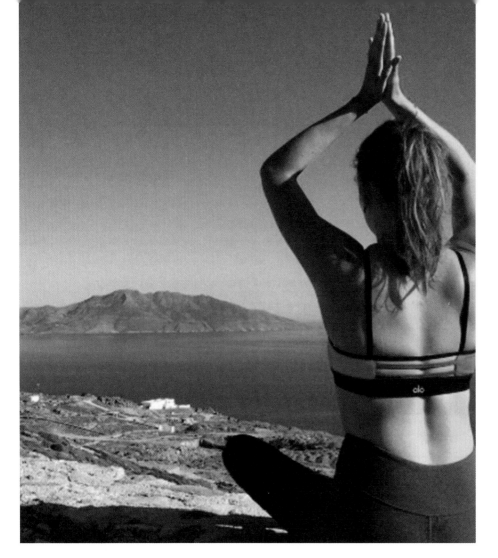

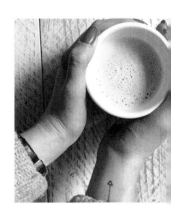

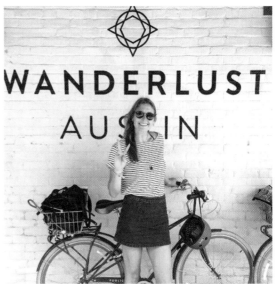

change in diet was really my starting point), my attitude towards other aspects of my life started to change, having a positive knock-on effect and driving me to create conditions for a truly healthy, happy lifestyle.

I have been, and continue to be, on a fascinating journey of self-discovery, learning a little more about myself every day. I have come to realize how powerful this knowledge is, and that it can really influence the many different parts of my life, allowing me to take decisions that nurture me. Most noticeably, I have learned to be kinder towards and more accepting of myself, something that so many of us find challenging. I still continue to learn and grow every day, and I hope that I will do so for ever. In the meantime, I want to share the power of this process and help guide you through all the confusing and conflicting information. I want to help you make sense of it all in a way that is manageable, that fits in with your life and allows you to really understand what it is that you need in order to find your own sense of balance.

Some of you might be reading this book because you are looking for a way to overcome a digestive disorder or low energy levels – or perhaps you've realized that you are not feeling as good as you would like. If this sounds familiar, then in many ways your motivation is probably already in place. You know why you are trying to make changes and can see how much your life could be improved if you can relieve yourself of whatever symptoms you are experiencing. However, when you try something and it doesn't work out, it can be incredibly frustrating – I know that from my own experience. For you, persevering when you can't find a quick fix may be challenging at times, but hopefully you will soon recognize the things that do and do not suit you.

Others of you perhaps might be a little curious, and even if you don't have a specific cause for immediate change, you might simply be interested in learning more about yourself or how to live life to the fullest. For you, making changes to your lifestyle can be harder to commit to, but perhaps a little less frustrating.

'Nothing about this book is intended to be prescriptive. The aim is to share with you a few ideas to help you work through your own journey, at a pace that suits you, in order to discover what makes you feel your absolute best.'

Alternatively, you may not fit in with either of those groups and maybe just picked this book up at random – if so, why not continue to flick through just a little longer and perhaps you'll spot something you like the look of, or a sentence or two that resonate with you? Whoever you are, taking the time to focus on yourself is a really positive exercise that can help you to get the most out of life, and hopefully help you to learn and grow in ways you might not have known you could.

I would never want to tell anyone how to approach their own life, but as you go through this book I would urge you to be open-minded, to step outside your comfort zone and go with the flow. Trial and error can be incredibly frustrating, but for most of us quick fixes just don't exist, especially if you are looking for long-term change. If you can find comfort in the idea that you are trying to do what is best for your mind and body, and that each day is a step towards figuring it all out, the whole process will become more manageable, no matter what setbacks you may face.

I hope this book serves as a guide for you. Nothing about it is intended to be prescriptive. The aim is to share a few ideas to help you work through your journey, at a pace that suits you. The most important thing to remember is that there is no right or wrong, no pass or fail.

This is all about you, learning about yourself and creating a life that allows you to feel your very best.

Another thing that I find so helpful to remember is that we are all insignificant. I mean this in the best possible way. Every time you face a problem that feels totally terrifying, take a step back and know that as much as you may think your actions will completely rock the world, they truly won't. Each of us, alone, is insignificant, but together we are a powerful force. Let's create individual consciousness on a large scale. Let's play, learn, grow and inspire the people around us. And most importantly, let's find ourselves, and learn to enjoy each moment, because nothing in life is permanent.

I want to show you how to fall in love with taking care of yourself – to help you navigate through the processes of connecting with yourself, and opening the door for you to walk through in order to find your own true balance.

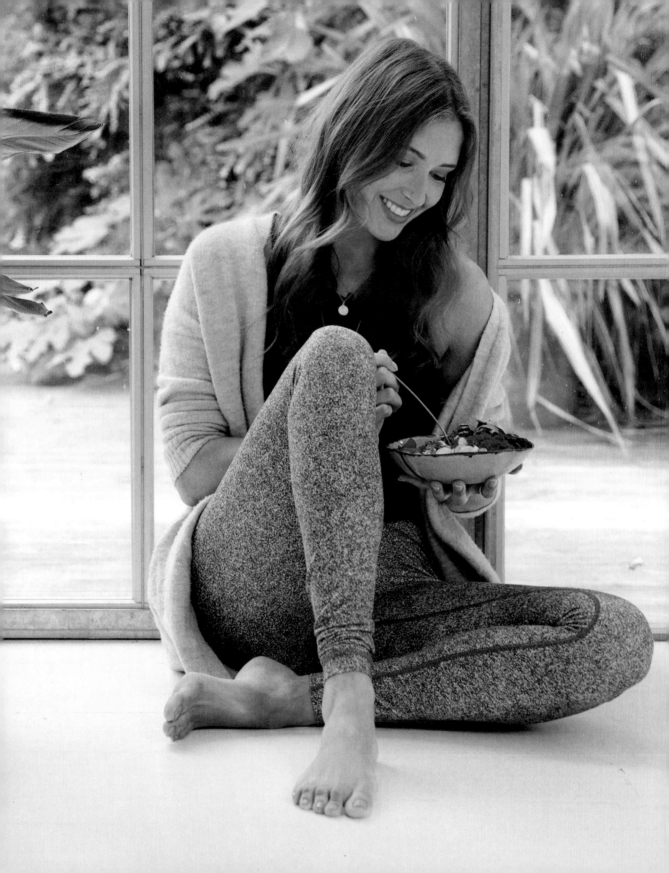

A bit of background

What I am sharing with you in this book is all stuff I learned on my journey to improve my physical and mental well-being.

You can draw inspiration from different theories, examples and other people's experiences, holding on to just the bits that work for you and letting go of the things that don't.

Throughout my teenage years, and especially as I got to university, I struggled a lot with both energy levels and digestive issues. Things seemed to get worse and worse until eventually I felt that it was having such an impact on my quality of life that I totally despaired. I remember calling my mum on an almost daily basis at a total loss about what to do. Every time I ate I was in so much discomfort, and not a moment went by that I wasn't aware of some sort of stomach-bloating after eating. I didn't even understand that it wasn't normal until my mum tried to get me to describe what I was feeling and I realized that other people didn't have this 24/7 digestive awareness. On top of all that, I got to the point where my body was seemingly so exhausted just trying to digest whatever I fed it that I couldn't physically stay awake after eating.

I eventually got to the point where I was so miserable that something really had to change. I decided to do a total 360-degree lifestyle turnaround and take out everything and anything from my diet that I thought could possibly cause any sort of stomach issues. I felt that structure would be really valuable to me, so I followed a strict high-protein diet, eating very simple meals based around chicken, turkey, eggs and fish, usually accompanied by brown rice and steamed veg. It was the sort of diet you would expect a body-builder to follow and, combined with some serious gym training to try to keep myself feeling strong and confident, I really bought into this rigid plan. I was in the best shape of my life: strong, fit and healthy, and for the first time in a long while I had the energy to get through each day again. My gut was almost healed, too – in fact, after just six weeks the improvement was so dramatic that I couldn't believe I had waited so long to make changes.

However, while I felt as though I had proved a miracle to myself in terms of my body, I began to struggle in other areas of my life. I was no longer drinking alcohol, and as a young adult in London whose friends had all started working in the City and many of whom were boozing their way from Wednesday to Sunday, I felt as though I was pretty isolated socially. My diet and newly discovered teetotal ways didn't go down particularly well in social situations, and often I would just choose not to go to that party, or dinner, or anything else due to a fear of the undesired attention I might draw.

I found that I developed a totally different lifestyle imbalance, whereby my quest for feeling good physically had caused me to shut myself away and lose out on quality time with the people I loved. I created space between me and my friends because although I was paying meticulous attention to making choices that made me feel good physically, I wasn't allowing myself to really relax in social situations. I didn't want to draw attention to myself by eating and drinking differently to everyone else, but I didn't want to sabotage all the progress I had made, either.

Over time I began to develop my understanding of true health and happiness as being so much more than just committing to a certain plan or regime created by someone else. While regimes absolutely served their purpose at points along my journey in helping to rid me of old habits, ultimately they were created for someone else with a different body and lifestyle from mine. Also, trying to stick to something so rigid led me, in the long run, to feel deprived in other areas of my life.

What I discovered was that you don't have to take an all-or-nothing approach, committing 100 per cent to taking what works for someone else and pasting it into your own life. You can draw inspiration from different theories, examples and other people's experiences, holding on to just the bits that work for you and letting go of the things that don't – without any guilt or feelings of failure.

As I became more in touch with my own body, I began to understand how to adapt to what it needed at different times. I began to think of being healthy as a dynamic process whereby different days, weeks, seasons and shifts in day-to-day activity levels, the weather and a hundred other factors affected how I felt, and that responding directly to how I was feeling was much more beneficial than adhering to some rigid plan just because I thought it was healthy. I found myself learning so much about how my own body responds to different foods and exercises that I was able to discover what makes me feel my best. The difficulty was sticking with things long enough to figure out what really made

a difference, and also accepting that even if something suits my body at a certain time, it doesn't mean it will a few months later. So, of course, it takes a lot of patience and trust that the entire process is ultimately a positive experience.

After outgrowing a job that I absolutely loved, I was a little lost about what to do with myself. I decided to qualify as a personal trainer as a way of earning a living. It made sense at the time as I had trained myself so much in the past that it seemed like a natural step. I wanted to share what I had learned, develop my own knowledge of the body and to help people build better relationships with themselves. I began training a few clients, which I enjoyed, but I didn't feel driven to become the best trainer I could be. I wanted to take on more clients, but didn't feel that I should be building new relationships when I wasn't 100 per cent committed. I needed to find a way to earn a living and decided that I was probably going to have to find myself a 'real' job. I had always wanted to do a yoga teacher training course to develop my own practice

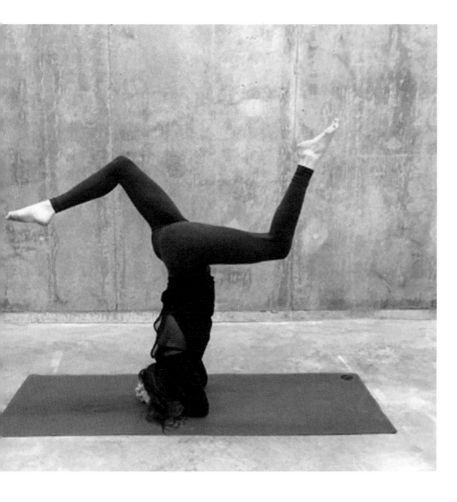

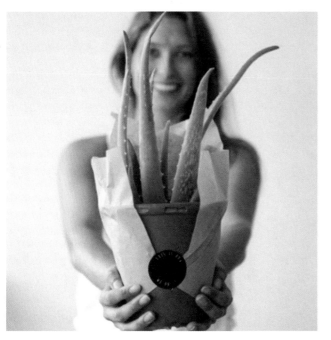

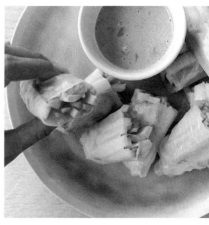

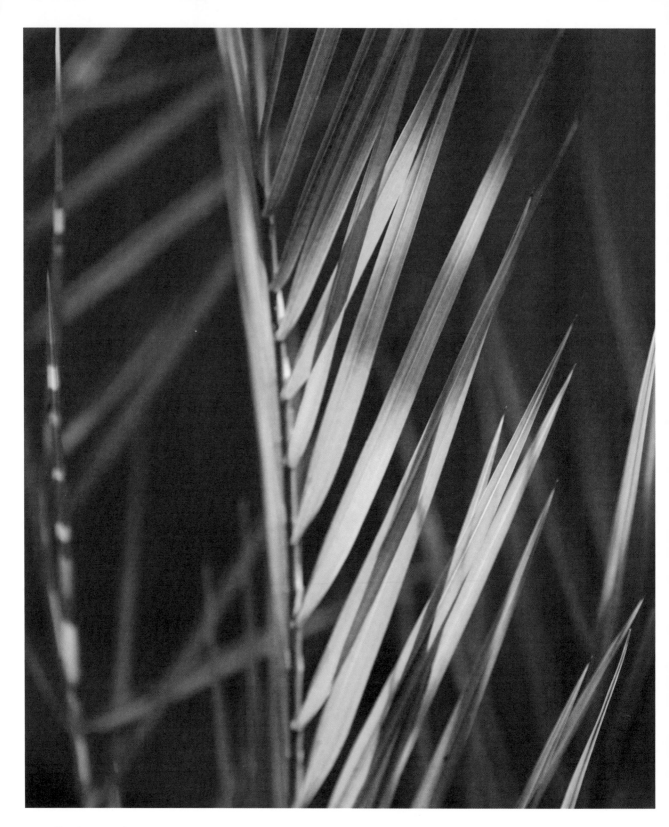

Background   20

'Understanding what works for you is an amazing skill to develop.'

and learn more about it, and so I decided to scrape together the last of my savings to take that time for myself before I got into the world of work where, inevitably, it would be a struggle to take a month out at any point in the foreseeable future. I booked a last-minute flight to Goa, India, and found a yoga school with a spare space in Agonda, South Goa.

As part of the training we started teaching just a few days in – and I finally realized I had found my thing. As clichéd as it sounds, for the first time in as long as I could remember I felt totally at home, comfortable, confident, calm and peaceful. Something about it seemed so natural to me and I loved every minute of

teaching from day one. I felt like I was creating a really wonderful connection with every student, and opening the door for them to connect with themselves. Facilitating that is one of the most wonderful things to watch. I really believe that I am offering them the key to something that they already have within themselves but don't know how to access. It is so moving to see how my students develop and grow, not just in their physical practice but also in the mental and emotional strength that they discover.

Becoming a teacher came at exactly the right moment. I really believe that all those occasions in the past when I had looked into doing a course and had decided for one reason or another not to do so was because it wasn't my time yet. To really give all that you can as a teacher takes a lot of hard work, and in my own experience with personal training I wasn't doing the right thing, or perhaps the timing wasn't right for having the necessary drive to develop myself in that direction. But a few short months later, with my qualification in hand, I felt – and still feel – driven to become the best yoga teacher I can be.

I was thrown in at the deep end with teaching, and I made a pact with myself to say 'yes' as often as possible to develop my teaching experience and to continue to learn and grow both as a teacher and as a student myself. I had to give myself a pep talk on many occasions to rid myself of the 'new teacher nerves' and find the confidence to accept opportunities with an open mind. Within two months of returning from India, I was teaching a room of sixty students for an event, and teaching more hours in a week than I expected to have done in the first few months. My confidence grew and I would bound out of bed at 5.30 a.m., ready for my first class or client of the day without a single thought of how anti-social the hour was! I was working seven days a week but it hardly felt like work. I was saying 'yes' to everything, keen to learn and put myself out there – and inevitably I ended up teaching a little too much. I was running around London all day to get to classes, meetings or whatever else I had scheduled. I had no time for my own practice, but was walking up to 20,000 steps a day and, despite eating (and eating) to fuel my busy days, weight seemed to just be dropping off me, which created a little concern for some of those close to me, and certainly was not my intention.

Within a few short weeks I was exhausted! My hips were killing me but I was loving every second of it and I didn't want to slow down. I soon came to realize that on top of my work with my blog, which was growing quickly and bringing its own opportunities, I couldn't sustain the pace if I wanted to look after my

'Most of the time I feel better than I ever knew I could: I have energy, I'm rarely stressed, I let things go and feel a lot less anxious … I am a lot more comfortable in my own skin.'

students and myself properly. I didn't want to miss an opportunity or let people down, but I quickly learned that to do something well takes commitment and time, and the more thinly I spread myself, the less likely I was to give my best. That was enough to encourage me to take a few steps back.

I always try to bring myself back to the reason why this all began. I started on this journey because I was trying to look after my own body and mind. If one of those, or both, becomes neglected then, within reason, I try to rein it in and see what can be done to find my balance again. Most of the time I feel better than I ever knew I could: I have energy, I'm rarely stressed, I let things go and feel a lot

less anxious. My stomach is generally much happier and I am a lot more comfortable in my own skin. I am still human and I am still learning. Sometimes my stomach plays up, or I have a week where I am feeling sluggish. There are still days when I don't feel so confident in myself. It is OK to feel that way sometimes, but I just try to remember not to indulge in it too much. You really can be so proactive in managing the way you feel; understanding what works for you is actually a really amazing skill to develop. It feels so wonderful to know that there is so much you can do to help yourself, so that even if you don't feel your best 100 per cent of the time, you can set yourself up for a pretty strong average.

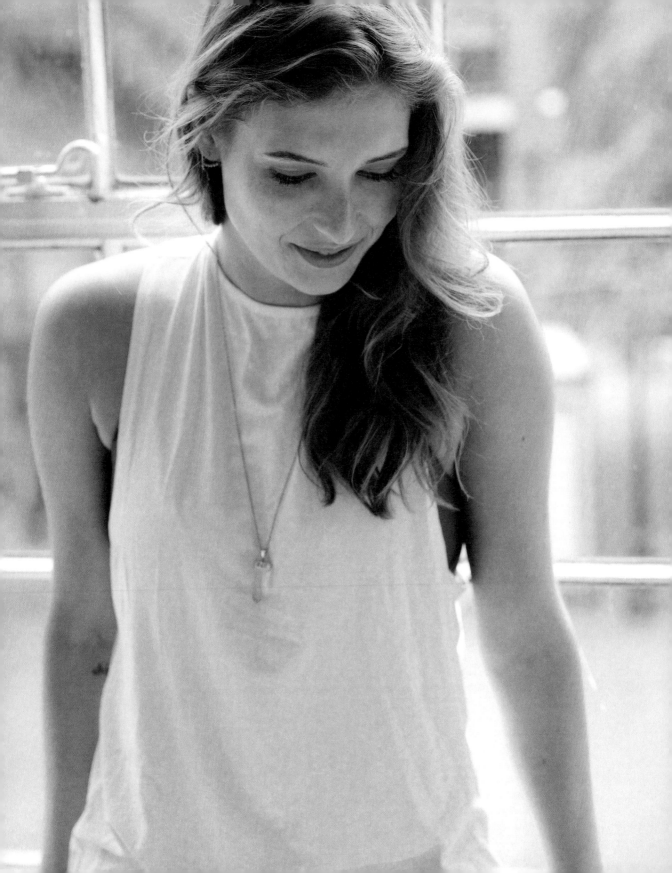

A few last words before we begin

Start from a place of positivity
and allow yourself the space
to grow and learn without
judgement or boundaries.

If you wait until you 'feel like it' every time you want to make a change, you might stay the same forever. Which is, of course, totally fine if you are happy where you are – but presumably the reason you've thought about doing something in the first place is because you feel you have something to gain from making that change.

I can't tell you the number of times I have sat down and meticulously planned a week so that I can get my work done, see all my clients, get to the gym and do my yoga practice, and been really excited to achieve it. But then it is Monday morning, or Tuesday afternoon, or any time in any day and I just don't feel like doing whatever is scheduled for that time. I remember that the washing needs doing or that I really must get through my emails, or that I 'need' to do absolutely anything else.

Whatever your goal is, you need to understand your motivation in order to be truly committed to achieving it. Rather than think you want to eat more healthily, be stronger, fitter, lose weight, spend more time with friends or whatever else it is that you are striving towards, take a step back and think about what you will gain by achieving it. For example, if you are hoping to lose weight, what will be the impact of that on your life? Perhaps it will improve your confidence or allow you to be more active? What are the results that will make a positive difference to you? Once you start to understand why you want to achieve something, you have a much greater level of motivation to spur you on if it gets tough at any point (and the chances are it will at times).

So often we resolve to make changes because there is something we don't like in our lives. The trouble is we then tell ourselves that we will be happy once we make this change.

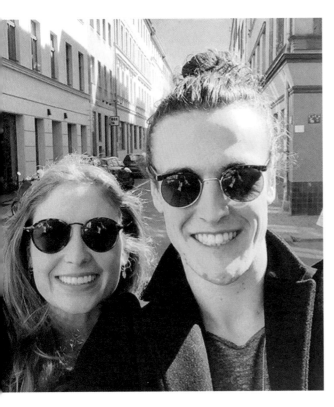

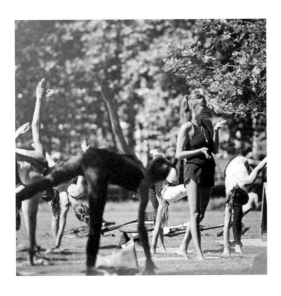

This mindset of changing because we don't like where we are poses a problem if we don't see results: it can be pretty frustrating and we bring ourselves down or feel as if we've failed if we don't get exactly where we wanted to be. If you can make a conscious decision to accept yourself first, everything shifts a little. It's so much more positive to make healthy changes to your lifestyle because you want to care for the amazing body and mind you have and look after them the best you can, than to make changes because you feel negative about yourself. It may be easier said than done, but it makes everything so much more manageable if you can accept yourself for who and where you are right now, before you embark on creating change.

Finally, allow yourself to be a beginner, to make mistakes, to figure out some things quickly and find other things much harder. Don't expect everything to fall into place straight away; in fact, try not to expect anything at all. This isn't about miracle cures or overnight success; it's about taking care of yourself, and learning exactly what you need.

Mind

— 01

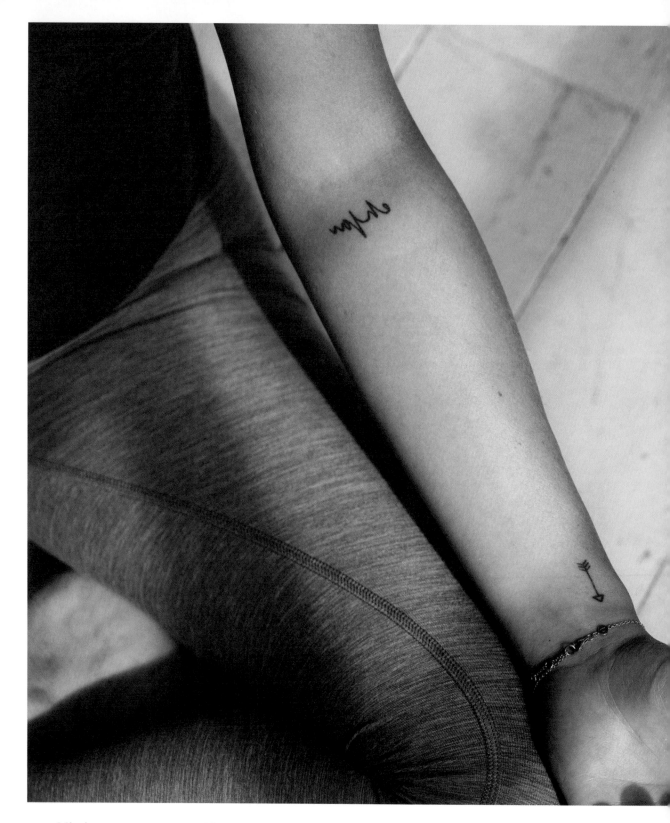

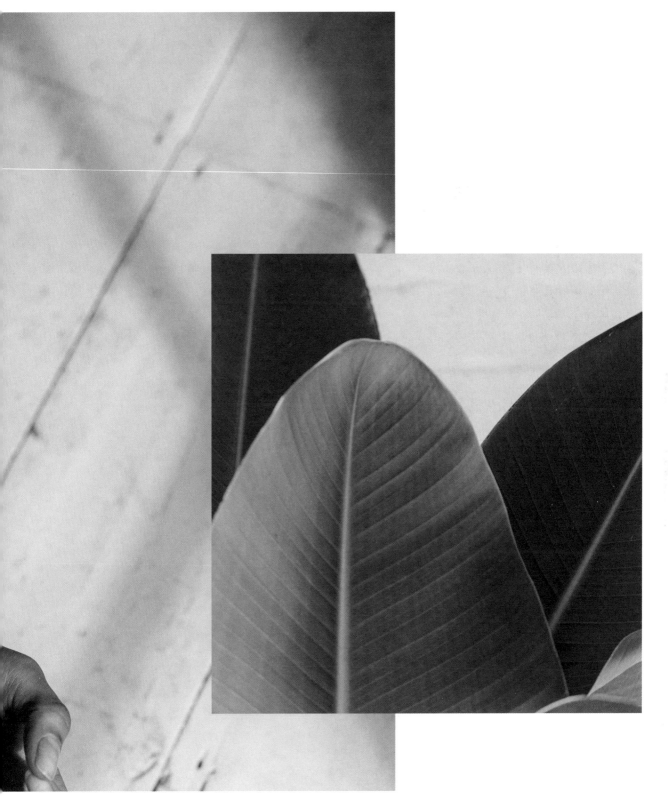

Like most of us, you probably go through each day without really noticing what you are thinking about.

Recently 'mindfulness' has become a bit of a buzzword and there are all sorts of programmes, apps and concepts that enable us to become more efficient in the workplace, develop a positive mentality and generally become happier. This can all seem a little strange if you didn't feel as though anything was 'wrong' in the first place. But no matter how comfortable you already are in your mind and thought processes, mindfulness can benefit all aspects of your life.

Your mind is a wonderfully complex thing, and each of our minds works in an individual way, making understanding others and ourselves a life-long adventure. For a lot

of people the mind ticks away without them really giving it any attention. Others may choose to try to understand a little more about how it works, how it influences their actions and how it is connected to the physical body, through practices such as yoga and meditation.

Put simply, being mindful means being aware of the present moment and having a conscious understanding and acceptance of the way you feel. I guess the thing to realize is that a mindfulness practice doesn't necessarily mean the same thing to each person. While some people consciously commit to a specific exercise to connect with themselves in a certain way, others may have a subconscious mindfulness practice that they include in their daily habits without even realizing or planning it.

As I shifted towards my current lifestyle and left old habits behind, I made a decision to accept that I can't predict where life will take me and I began to think more deeply about what I really wanted. I came to the conclusion that I wanted to be two things – healthy and happy – to give myself the best chance of coping with and enjoying the twists and turns of the future. So what did I need to do to equip myself to deal with whatever might come my way? What did being truly happy mean? What constituted health? Did that include my mental health as well as healthy attitudes? Suddenly there were a million things to consider and it all seemed fairly complicated.

As these thoughts developed, I asked myself what really makes me happy. I realized that, like many people, I often associated happiness with something that I didn't have. Most of us probably set goals in our lives such as promotions, aesthetic triumphs or other personal and professional achievements, and we tell ourselves that when we've reached them we'll be happy. In reality, it seems to be that when we do reach a goal, we have already found something else to focus on, shifting the goalposts again. It is so easy to end up in a cycle of chasing happiness, but never allowing ourselves to reach it. I've seen it in myself. I guess it's a little like the saying 'the grass is always greener' – if we condition happiness on a future state, there is always going to be something else to achieve, meaning that happiness is indefinitely out of reach.

For many people, setting goals is a tool for self-development – but you have to be wary about resting your happiness on achieving goals. If you constantly chase an end goal, you lose out on so many days of feeling fulfilled by where you are right now. You have to reframe your thinking in order to find happiness on the way towards your goals. It is also necessary to appreciate that you are not in total control: sometimes you can have your heart set on something that is, due to external factors, simply unachievable.

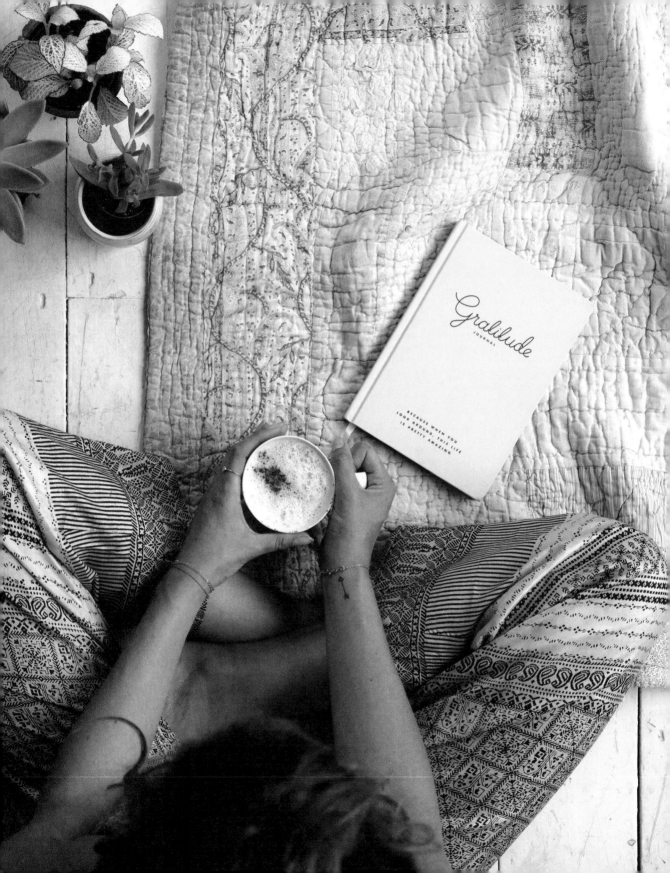

Being Present

You know when you are having a conversation with someone and they are there physically but they're not really 'there'? They're reading something or watching something, or they're otherwise focused so they can hear what you are saying, and may even be responding, but they're not actually listening. I always notice this and try hard not to take offence. I remind myself that I should try never to do this to someone else. However, in truth, I know that sometimes I can be that person, too.

Think how often you are sitting with a friend and your phone beeps on the table in front of you. You distract yourself for a moment by looking at your phone and suddenly you are caught up in a totally different conversation. You might still be engaging with the person you are with, but are you really being present? How much of your attention are you really giving that person?

I remember vowing to commit fully to the company I'm in as much as possible after a friend once commented on my lack of attention on one particular occasion. It stuck with me, and while there are, of course, still times when I don't manage to keep it up totally, I have come up with a few things that I find make it easier to give my attention more fully to the physical (as opposed to virtual) company I'm in.

It is OK to be busy. If you are meeting a friend and an email needs to be sent in order to prevent your mind from wandering mid-conversation, try saying something like, 'Bear with me just two minutes and then you have my full attention,' and really mean it. Everyone deserves undivided attention, but especially after politely waiting for you to get whatever needs to be addressed out of the way in order to follow through with your statement of commitment.

If you are in the above situation and there is a call that you really cannot miss or delay, then make that known to the person you are with from the beginning. If you tell them that you are expecting an important call and ask if they mind if you slip away to answer it, then at least you have shown them some consideration.

Most of us spend so much time with our phones glued to our hands. All it takes is a flick of the eyes towards your screen mid-meeting and you can lose your train of thought, and you appear disinterested in your immediate company. Whenever you are in the presence of another person (socially, for work or otherwise), keeping your phone away from the table is a really easy way to avoid distraction.

Be Kind – Starting with Yourself

We need to get out of the negative mindset where we tell ourselves we aren't good enough, don't look or feel good enough, don't try hard enough, and so on. People are often a lot more cruel to themselves than they would ever dream of being to other people. We spend so much time criticizing ourselves, and this can really intensify negative subconscious thought processes.

If you think about the pep talks you give your friends when they have their confidence knocked, or all the lovely things you might say to someone else – well, you deserve to hear those things, too. It is a huge step for a lot of people, but if you can find a way to be kinder to yourself, it can make a huge difference to how you see and cope with certain situations.

Of course, there are many ways you can show yourself kindness, and how we look after our bodies and minds is a big part of this.

Tools such as yoga and meditation can be a really great way not only to take care of yourself but also to delve a little deeper into understanding what you can do for yourself.

For example, there are two sets of ethical values in yoga, known as the Yamas and the Niyamas, which offer moral codes to live by. The first of the Yamas is Ahimsa, or non-violence. Yoga is a non-violent practice but sometimes we try to push ourselves or get frustrated within our practice. Letting go of expectation and judgement of ourselves and approaching our practice with kindness and compassion is learning to adopt the concept of Ahimsa.

This is something that we can then apply to other areas of our lives. It seems so obvious to practise non-violence towards other people or beings, but how often do we include ourselves in this?

'It is so incredibly freeing to let go of expectation and judgement towards yourself and to truly accept every part of your being.'

As soon as you start being kinder to yourself, you can alleviate some of the negativity that can so easily dampen your true nature. It is incredibly freeing to let go of expectation and judgement towards yourself and to truly accept every part of your being. I imagine there are few people who can say they have detached entirely from personal criticism. But it isn't about being perfect; it is much more about taking steps towards acceptance in order to help us to grow as individuals.

Comparing ourselves to others is the root of so much social anxiety. One of the things I am learning is that the world of social media really is a crazy one. On the one hand, it gives us the opportunity to connect with a broad number of people from all over the world, and opens us up to new ideas and sources of inspiration. On the other hand, we are then exposed to all of these people whose profiles aren't necessarily a true reflection of reality. It is inevitable that we then have feelings of insecurity or dissatisfaction with our own lives, when compared to enhanced versions of other people.

The best person to compare yourself to is surely yourself. Rather than trying to match up to someone else, being the best version of you is such a wonderful way to focus your energy. Accepting who you are and focusing on that rather than on comparing yourself to others can be a healthy and positive thing to work on.

Learning to Look Out for Number One

Many of us spend our whole lives worrying about others, trying to fix their problems and even taking responsibility for the happiness of friends and family. However, taking the weight of others on your shoulders can cause you to overlook taking care of yourself.

We are all responsible for our own happiness and we have to find it within ourselves, rather than constantly search for it in external sources. In the same way, while you can have a positive impact on other people you cannot take responsibility for someone else's happiness. They hold that responsibility themselves. So in a sense you have to learn to become a little bit selfish and ensure that you get enough of what you need to be content in your life.

The question arises, then, of what it is that you want. And that's where tuning in with yourself is crucial, because there is so much to learn about ourselves that we can only find out by connecting with who we really are.

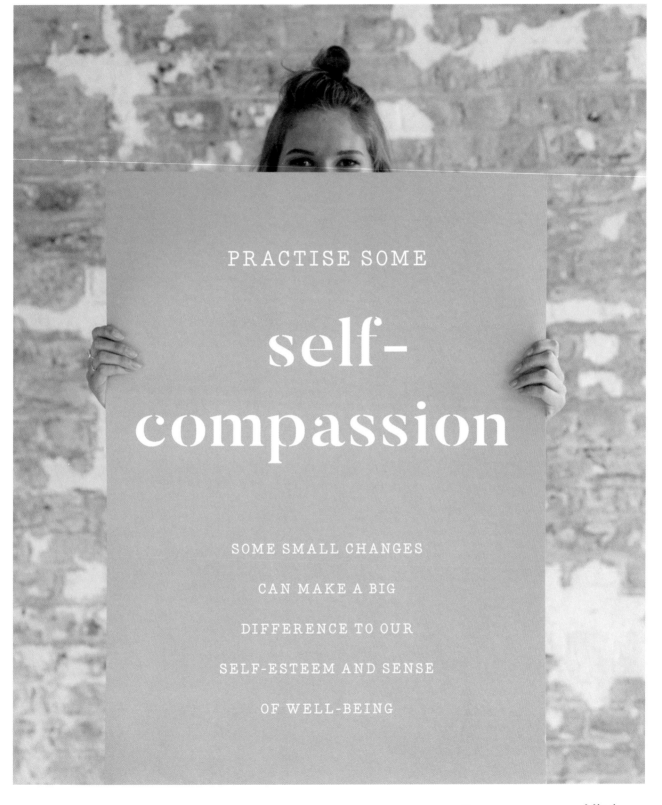

PRACTISE SOME

self-compassion

SOME SMALL CHANGES

CAN MAKE A BIG

DIFFERENCE TO OUR

SELF-ESTEEM AND SENSE

OF WELL-BEING

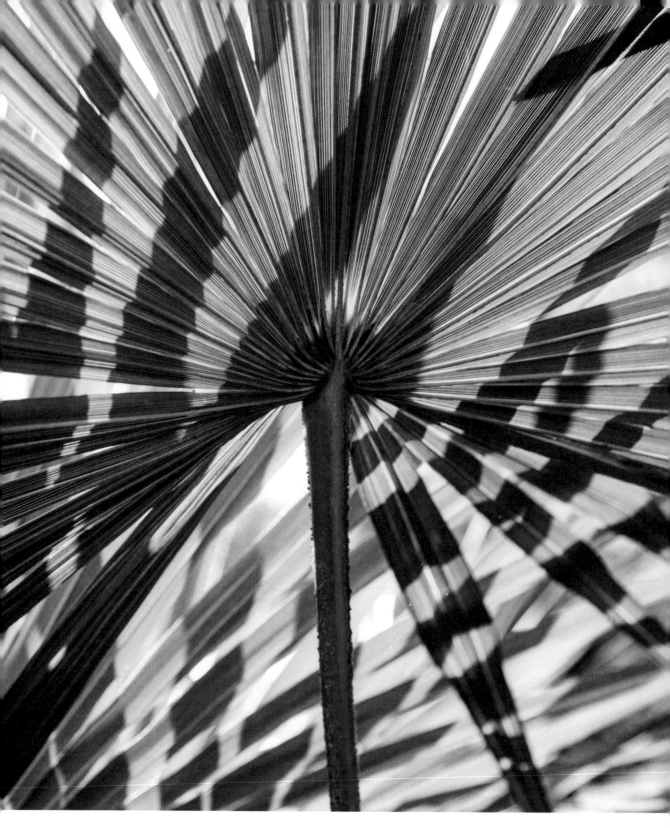

The Reality of it All

For most people, a lifestyle that revolves entirely around a passion may not be totally feasible. With greater responsibility generally comes less flexibility, and any risk becomes much greater. Whatever you've committed to that is preventing you from taking a leap now, there are still so many ways in which you can adapt your lifestyle to find a better balance.

For some people, their job is their passion. For others it might just be a means to an end. Most of us spend such a big part of our lives working, so being able to find the positive in each day can go a long way towards making us happy. Of course, we can't all run off and do what we would love to do all day every day – and even those who love what they do have

'If you can find a way to do as much of what you love as possible, you allow yourself the opportunity to live a more fulfilling, happier lifestyle.'

their ups and downs – but if you can find a way to do as much of what you love as possible, you allow yourself the opportunity to live a more fulfilling, happier lifestyle.

We all take pleasure from different things. Some people are motivated to earn a good salary, perhaps so that they can take more expensive holidays, for example; others might be more inclined to live a simpler life if it means they have more time to enjoy the things they love. Someone with expensive hobbies may be happy to work longer hours, so they can afford to do the things they enjoy more in their time off. Some people like to feel amazing all the time, and so commit to a healthy, wholesome lifestyle; others may prefer to dip in and out of healthy choices, choosing to party or do the things they really enjoy without concern of whether or not it is good for them because it makes them feel good in other ways. Different things make each of us tick, and the best thing you can do for yourself is to indulge in whatever you enjoy whenever you can (within reason) and find your balance.

It can be hard to determine what these things really are, but there are fundamental questions you can ask yourself that might make things clearer. By taking the time to sit down and answer them honestly and fully, you can take stock of what you truly want from life.

When you are eighty or ninety years old and looking back on your life, **what would you like to have seen, done and learned?**

Does what you're doing now, day to day, **allow you** to do those things?

If you were totally free from responsibility (financial or otherwise), **how would you spend your time?**

What makes you happy that already exists in your life?

What makes you unhappy?

When do you feel **completely yourself?**

What do you **value?**

Who do you **value** and why?

Why do you do the things that you do?

Why do you hold **certain opinions and attitudes?** Are they true to you and what you really believe?

It's easy to look at these questions and come up with superficial answers, but when you take time to think a little more deeply it can be a very helpful exercise in developing an understanding of yourself and your values. Of course, this is not an exhaustive list of things to reflect upon, but it can serve as a first step towards creating a more balanced lifestyle. Most of us are creatures of habit and sometimes we have to actively examine – and even disrupt – our normal thought and behavioural patterns in order to recognize what we really want and need.

When you spend lots of time with someone who has a different accent to you, you might find that you pick up a little of their intonation or speech patterns. They are not your own, they are just adopted from the environment that you have been in. I'm particularly susceptible to acquiring accents – I've never known why, or if there is some sort of psychology behind it, but it has certainly caused a few giggles at my expense!

This applies to more than just how you speak. When you spend a lot of time with other people or in certain environments, sometimes their opinions, traits, habits and attitudes can make your own values a little hazy. Sometimes this will help you to develop your own values and sometimes there will be layers and layers of these 'inherited' behaviours and thoughts to remove in order to get back to being truly yourself.

What habits or opinions have you collected along the way? Being influenced by people around us helps to shape who we are, and often this can be for the better, but we need to examine these attitudes to make sure we are still being true to ourselves.

Learning to connect with yourself is probably not the sort of thing you can learn overnight. In fact, I don't know if we ever can know ourselves entirely – or at least that is not yet within my own experience – but you can certainly do things to encourage the process, and it can be a wonderful and interesting journey.

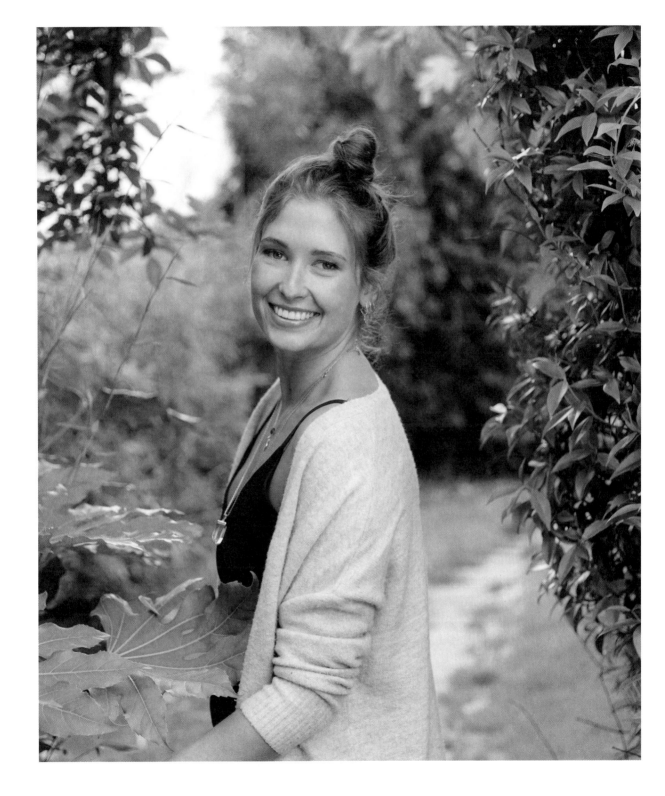

Mind

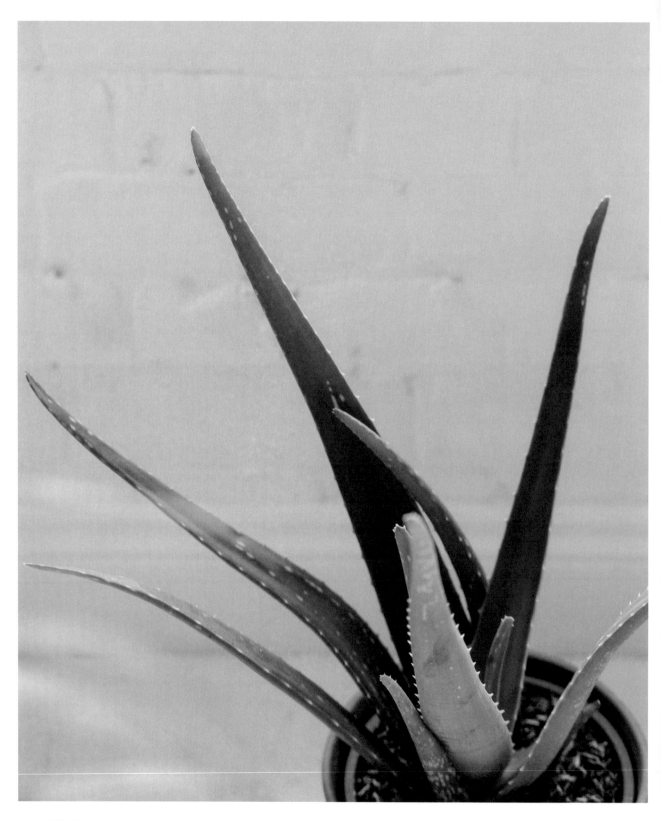

Understanding
Your Feelings

Emotions are something that we all experience in different ways. For some of us, showing our emotions comes more naturally than for others, and there is no right or wrong way to deal with the twists and turns of life. People talk about being 'emotionally intelligent'; having the ability to understand both your own and other people's emotional behaviour. We are all wired so differently that the way you react to a situation, or the way that something or someone makes you feel, shouldn't be classed as right or wrong. What is important is to recognize these differences in order to connect with both yourself and other people.

Being mindful about our emotions allows us to alter the way we behave in future situations.

There is a lesson to learn from everything, and all emotions serve a positive purpose. Sensitivity is wonderful if it means that you are able to read situations and evaluate responses. Providing other people with a map to read us helps them to understand how best to support us in our times of need. Of course, understanding yourself better allows you to rationalize your emotions, making life a little less turbulent than it might otherwise be.

No matter how you deal with things, it isn't about good or bad, but just how you are. You need to accept the way in which you and those around you deal with things, embrace the highs and lows, learn from them and release any judgement and frustration that they may bring.

Managing the Mind

The difficulty with any sort of mindfulness practice or mind exercise is that the results aren't tangible in the same way that other lifestyle changes are. There are no 'before' and 'after' photos, nor a number on the scales to go by, so it can be difficult to really understand what is and isn't working for you.

Becoming ever more conscious of yourself and switching away from living on auto-pilot allows you to be more in touch with who you really are and know what you truly value, enabling you to take steps in the direction that serves you best.

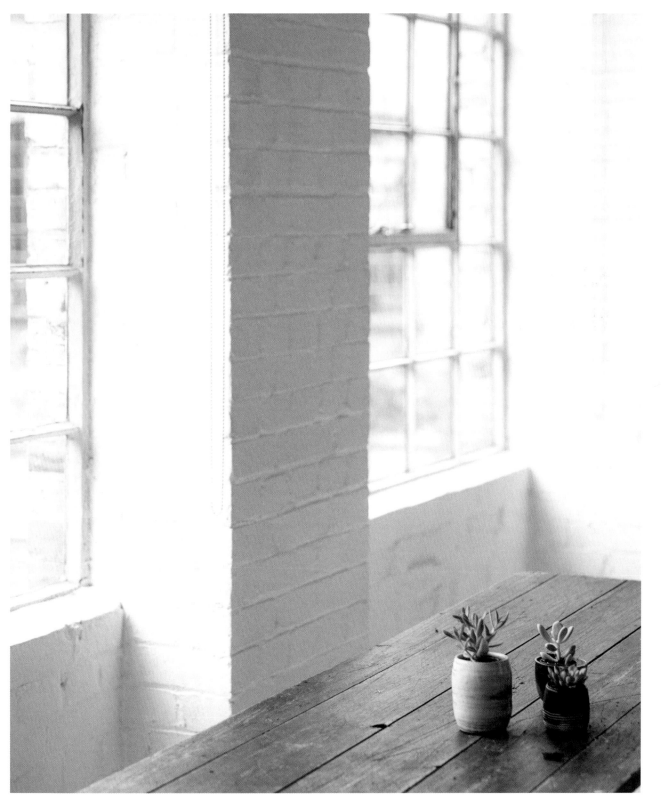

As an adult I have become more and more aware of the number of people who experience symptoms of anxiety or depression to some degree or at certain periods in their lives. I don't know if it is because people are becoming more open, life is becoming more stressful, or perhaps there are just more people who have the courage to identify themselves as having these struggles, but I find it interesting to consider what leads so many of us down this path, and if there is anything we can do or change to prevent it having such an impact on our minds.

I think many of us try to take responsibility for things that are beyond our control, and as a result experience guilt or other emotions that cause stress and anxiety to build up in our minds. I'm one of those people who takes the weight of everyone else's problems on my shoulders as my own, without being asked, and I have begun to realize that I feel very guilty about things that are not in my power. So much is ultimately beyond our control and sometimes we just have to let go of that need or desire to solve problems. I have had to learn that I can still be a good friend without knowing all the answers, and that it is OK to put myself first at times.

Worry is another emotion that I find cripples a lot of people and prevents them enjoying the moment. When you worry about the future, you are encouraging your fears to manifest in reality. We can help ourselves by trying to shift away from that focus on the uncertainty of things to come.

You have the power to choose how you feel and react. Of course, emotions are natural and your initial response to a situation may seem beyond your control – but if you take a step back, you can recognize that you have the power to choose. If you can learn not to be at the mercy of circumstance, and instead find a positive in every situation in which you find yourself, you will lighten the load you carry.

Fitting positivity into your day doesn't have to be time-consuming or challenging. There are simple things you can do to break negative thought patterns or reframe difficult parts of your day. Gratitude exercises can

'Of course, it is much easier to come up with a list of things you are grateful for when you have had a great day and things feel as though they are going well, but it is even more valuable when the words don't come quite so easily.'

be really helpful, for example. Often it can feel easier to focus on the small proportion of negative instead of the large proportion of positive, so by starting a gratitude journal, you can begin to shift this balance.

Even if the concept of writing down the things you are thankful for sounds a little odd, making a note of a few things when you wake up or before you fall asleep allows you to step back and reflect on the day without being caught up in the immediate moment. Of course, it is much easier to come up with a list of things you are grateful for when you have had a great day and things feel as though they are going well, but it is even more valuable when

the words don't come quite so easily. It is those days when you have to reframe the way you are thinking that can prove most uplifting. Repeating the practice on a daily basis can really help to train the mind to think more positively and can change how you approach your day-to-day life.

A lot comes down to acceptance – acknowledging that not everything will always go just the way you'd hoped, but can still be appreciated for what it is, for the challenges it gives you. Gratitude allows you to navigate each day with a more positive mindset, which helps you to enjoy the journey rather than just anticipate the outcome.

Embrace Imperfection

Negative talk about yourself or other people can be totally emotionally draining. I realized while I was doing my yoga teacher-training how much of an impact it had on me when one of my peers persistently criticized various aspects of the training. It was really wearing me down, and I eventually asked the group if we could try to go for a day without judging or criticizing, and just accept that we all may like and dislike different things but that it was all part of the journey we were on. I was really surprised by how strongly my energy could be affected by the negative talk of others, and I realized that not participating in that sort of conversation, or taking myself out of that situation, could reduce that impact.

'Finding a more positive way to think about who you are and what you do feeds a positive, creative energy that allows you to grow.'

In doing so I found such a positive relief, and I was able to maintain a more optimistic outlook and surrender to the full experience.

It can be invaluable to embrace every imperfection in your being and in the world around you. We will inevitably all have moments when we worry about what people think, when we criticize our progress, our bodies, our work, or doubt ourselves in any number of ways, but it is so freeing to accept that, firstly, it is OK not to be the finished article yet, and secondly, that imperfection is what makes us unique. Every quirk in our being is what makes us truly ourselves.

This all links back to the way that we talk to ourselves. Finding a more positive way to think about who you are and what you do feeds the positive, creative energy that allows you to grow. It's not just about shifting away from or trying to change what you don't like about yourself, but actually choosing to enjoy those imperfections as part of who you are, and accepting that they are a key part of you.

The same thinking can be applied to how situations play out in the world around you. Lots of us like to plan, idealize or predict how things might happen, but in reality our expectations may not be met or perhaps are exceeded. Rather than feeling disappointed, let down or overwhelmed by any outcome, you can choose how to react and make peace with a situation for just being what it is.

Stress Management

We live in a world surrounded by stress. I realized a little while ago that whenever I bumped into someone and we did that quick, 'Oh hi, how are you? How is work?', etc. that the answer I gave was always, 'Busy. Good but busy,' but what I really meant was 'I'm feeling pretty stressed!'. And their response was normally the same. I was telling the truth and so were they, but the monotony of it all started to bother me. Being busy is a transient state (even if it feels never-ending at times), but it doesn't define how we are as human beings.

Putting Off Tasks
Just Prolongs Them

One of my worst habits is flagging emails. I will have every intention of replying but so often I read something, become distracted without replying and flag it for later so that my focus shifts away from my ever-expanding inbox. It isn't productive or helpful; it is just setting myself up for a stressful time trying to clear it later.

This kind of procrastination is so futile. Putting off smaller tasks leaves them hanging over you. Instead of flagging emails or leaving the chores that you don't want to do until last, getting them done and ticking them off the list is such a simple step that can have a positive impact on the rest of your day. If there is something you really dislike or even dread, perhaps try to get it out of the way so that you no longer have to worry about it. You will immediately feel more accomplished. It sounds easy and, of course, is much more easily said than done – it can certainly take a lot of will-power, but it really is an incredibly positive habit to get into.

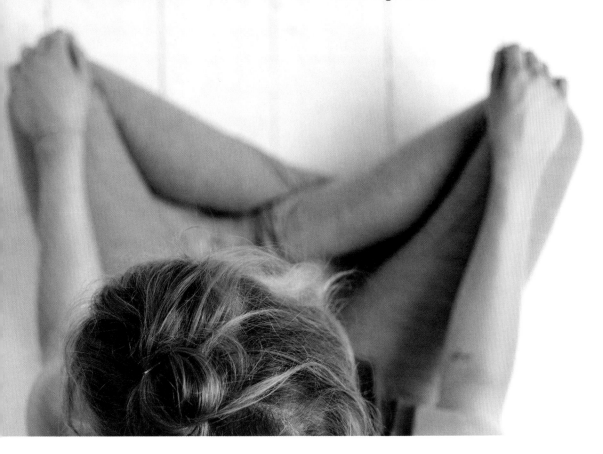

TO CREATE A

positive
attitude

AND ATTRACT POSITIVE

THINGS IN OUR LIVES,

WE HAVE TO RELEASE WHAT

DOESN'T SERVE US

Letting Go

People used to tell me that I forgive too easily. I've never been able to hold a grudge. I can't sleep on an unresolved disagreement or leave somewhere without making peace with whoever I'm leaving. I'd never really thought about it much, but I just don't seem to have any need or desire for that sort of tension or animosity, as I end up riddled with an over-dramatic feeling of guilt. But everyone is wired differently and for some people it is a lot harder to let go of something that has upset or frustrated them.

A middle ground is perhaps a really good place to be. If you can't forgive, you are holding on to anger, tension and emotions that can become toxic in your body and mind. So you are the one who ultimately suffers. Of course there's a fine line, and someone who forgives easily runs the risk of being walked all over or losing out by taking the emotional hit from a situation, but as long as you learn to differentiate between the two, it can be so freeing to let go of negative emotions that weigh you down.

I truly believe that holding onto frustration, anger or a need to control ultimately only leaves us being the one who loses out.

Breathing and Pranayama

Breath work is one of the most powerful tools we have. It can be linked to emotion, energy, well-being and our state of mind. In yogic philosophy, the breath (or prana) is seen as the life-force, yet most of us rarely take a moment to consider it.

Breath control, known in yoga as pranayama, can be used to calm the mind and help shift the way you approach your life. It allows you to take the first step towards mindfulness and meditation practices, so it can be particularly useful for those intimidated by traditional meditation techniques.

Breath work alone can have a huge impact on how you feel. I have found it a very powerful tool in times of stress, anxiety or whenever I have felt overwhelmed by life in general. I've even read that it can even help to reduce things like stress-induced overeating, by providing an alternative, calming focal point.

There are many different pranayama exercises that you can practise, but the most simple is known as abdominal breathing and it is a great starting point. It's an exercise that draws your awareness towards the breath. Focusing your attention on each inhalation and exhalation can help to still a busy mind, making this technique great for times of anxiety or just to help you relax at the end of a busy day.

I find it useful as a way to quieten my thoughts, reset my mind and find a more calm and rational approach to whatever challenge I am facing. It can also be used as a gentle energizer if I am feeling sluggish or sleepy. There is no need to have a 'sacred' space for this – in fact, it is good to practise non-attachment by trying different spaces for your yoga, meditation and pranayama, so just find a place where you can relax, sit comfortably and avoid distractions. It is generally not recommended to meditate lying down. Meditation allows you to enter a deeply relaxing state similar to sleep, so sitting up helps you to stay conscious.

Sit comfortably on the floor, or if you are in a chair then keep your legs uncrossed. Ensure that your spine is straight and your head is facing forward.

Begin by closing your eyes.

Take a few natural breaths here without trying to change anything at all. Just observe the breath within your body.

Become aware of each inhale and exhale, noticing if the breath is shallow or deep, and perhaps starting to tune in to any tightness or blockages within your body as the air passes in and out.

Closing your mouth, breathing only through your nose, consciously start to deepen each breath – inhale for a count of four, hold for one count, then exhale for a count of four. Hold for one count with empty lungs, then repeat. You can begin to lengthen the counts, perhaps to six or eight, and really try to draw your awareness to the sensation of the breath as it moves in and out of your body. If any thoughts come into your mind, just let them pass through without judgement or deliberation, allowing yourself to come back to the breath.

You can continue this practice for as long as you like, but five to ten minutes is a great length of time to work with.

Meditation

Breath-control exercises such as the one on the previous page are a wonderful way to start developing a meditation practice, if that is something that you want to try. Meditation can be an incredible tool for managing anxiety, depression, stress or just to help us generally in our day-to-day lives. At first I was a little nervous about the concept – as someone who spent the majority of my life unable to sit still for more than thirty seconds, I assumed it would never be for me. The idea of sitting on my own in silence was terrifying. For many of us it can be very difficult to control our minds and we have particular thought patterns that can be triggered by everyday events; for some of us this can contribute to stress and anxiety, or fluctuations in our moods. Even if we feel pretty happy most of the time, of course, some things can throw us occasionally.

The more you understand yourself and the way your mind works, the better equipped you are to deal with difficult things that may arise. Meditation is a powerful tool, as it helps you to understand yourself and provides you with a technique to guide your thoughts and condition the mind to cultivate positivity, not just during meditation practice but in the rest of your day, too.

One of the biggest challenges of meditation is creating the time for it. When you are stressed and busy, taking time out to meditate can seem counter-intuitive, but meditation can take a number of different forms, and although there are some specific styles of traditional meditation, you can really make anything your meditation if you choose. It's about finding time to be totally present, perhaps with a focus on the breath, and just tuning in to your mind and body. This could be

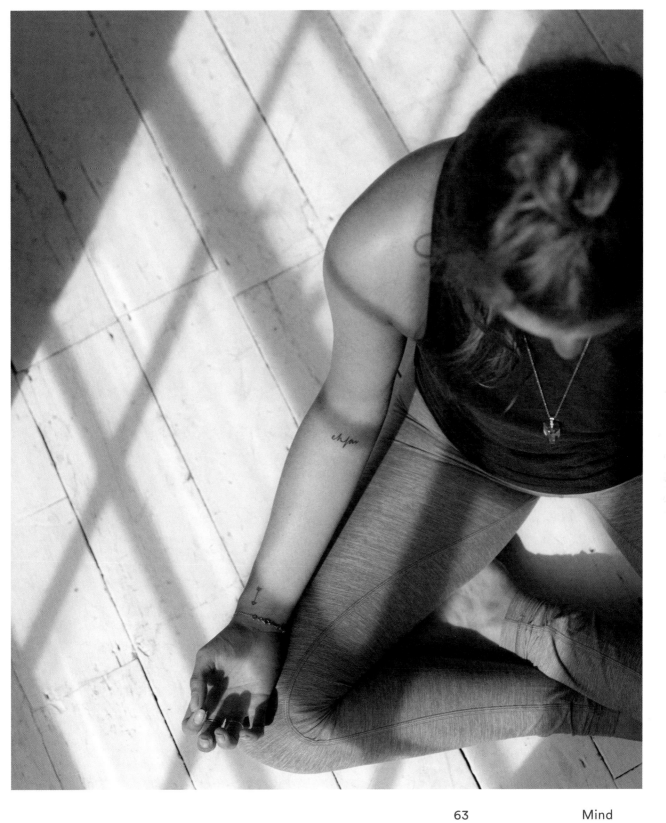

walking the dog, for example – anything that gives you some space. You can begin to develop a meditation practice at home, using various techniques or guides. There are some fantastic apps that give a very structured approach to building meditation or mindfulness into your everyday life. Some use guided meditations, where you are given a sound recording of someone speaking in order to direct your thoughts. Others are designed to encourage a more personal practice, perhaps giving you a certain thing to think about, and then setting a certain time frame, in order for you to develop that process individually.

Which approach is the best to use is so personal that it is almost impossible to give a recommendation. I would encourage you to explore the different options available, choose one that resonates the most and commit to it for a certain period of time. The reason I suggest this is because meditation is incredibly difficult. The first time, the first few times or the first hundred times, might be so challenging that you feel you are unable to turn off the busy-ness of the mind in any way at all. That in itself can lead to anxiety or discourage you from trying again. Remember that a strong meditation or mindfulness practice is not something that comes overnight. It is a continuous and indefinite process of connecting with yourself and removing any interruptions that you may encounter in your head.

Over time – slowly for some, more quickly for others – you will begin to notice that this starts to become ever so slightly easier and a committed practice can help in many areas of your life. The problem with something like meditation, as opposed to fitness, for example, is that there are no real tangible results as such, so if you are results-driven it takes a slight shift in perspective to notice the changes that meditation can produce.

If you're not sold on the idea of meditation, how about just working with being present? When was the last time you went about routine activities with a totally present mind? I know that I usually use the time

'At first meditation can be a lot harder than you might think, but it is a really valuable practice that helps you to become more present in your actions and spend less time on auto-pilot.'

brushing my teeth, showering or doing the washing up to list what needs to be done that day, plan ahead and go over thoughts and unresolved issues – and these repetitive thought patterns can be totally exhausting. Rather than focusing on other things, try to focus all your senses when you're doing something you do every day. It doesn't have to be showering. It could be eating breakfast, spending time with a friend or anything else.

When someone first asked me if I was interested in meditation I had a very naïve impression of what it actually was. I was so sure that meditation would never be for me. I liked people, distractions, noise and a fast pace of life. I didn't understand the benefits,

and to be honest I wasn't interested. It is so funny now to think back to how I viewed things not so many years ago, and how much more open I now am to new suggestions.

I suppose yoga introduced me to meditation without me ever realizing it. Breathing techniques and simple guided meditations in some classes meant that I was experiencing meditation without even knowing it. So when I was later introduced to it more formally, I was much more open-minded.

I considered going on an intensive weekend to learn how to meditate, but I could never justify the cost or commit to the time. I think we can always find an excuse if we want to. I continued to try meditation sessions on an ad hoc basis. I remember going into my first one, an hour-long session with around forty people. As I was arriving I told myself to be open-minded and that the worst that could happen would be that I had to sit in silence planning whatever I had coming up that week. In actual fact, the time passed in an instant and I left feeling energized and proud of myself. So I continued to dip in and out on a very non-committal basis for a year or so. I then went away to do my yoga teacher-training where we were introduced to various meditation techniques over the course of a month, meditating for thirty to sixty minutes a day, and after experimenting with different methods I grew quite fond of the early morning ritual.

Of course, I came back to London and didn't manage to keep it up for more than a few days, despite my best intentions. My diary was hectic and there was always something else that took priority. I was craving the calm and the headspace but not allowing myself it.

I was then invited to join an intensive Vedic meditation, a ten-hour introduction split into four sessions, the first of which was an hour-long initiation where we were given a personal mantra (a sound upon which we were taught to meditate). Within moments I had slipped into a deep state of consciousness and was pretty excited by how easy it had been. I was asked to try to do the same thing at home the next morning and, despite the ease of the previous day's practice, I just could not get my mind to switch off, so I arrived that evening at the group session with lots of questions. We then discussed the feelings and sensations that can be experienced before we went on to meditate individually, but still in this group environment, for twenty minutes. When I opened my eyes I was totally wiped, white as a ghost and overwhelmed by the experience. I was confused by how different each meditation seemed, but excited to learn more. Again, we were set the task of a home meditation before reconvening the next day and, just like before, I couldn't seem to get into it at home. Having felt so emotionally unstable and drained of all energy the previous evening, I was a little apprehensive of what was to come, but later that morning in the group session I had a totally energizing meditation which threw me even more, teaching me a valuable lesson on releasing expectations around the subject and just allowing myself to go with the flow.

What I hope my experience here shows is that sometimes we aren't ready to try something just yet, and perhaps we won't fully benefit from an experience if we force ourselves to do it at a certain time. However, there is a balance between waiting for the right time and taking a leap out of our comfort zone to explore what could be a really amazing thing.

My meditation practice now doesn't fall into a particular style or format; I have taken what I have learned from my various teachers and adapted it to work for me. And no, it doesn't happen every single day, despite my best intentions. But that is OK, too – it is all a dynamic and ongoing journey.

Meditation can seem a scary concept. If you are not ready to try traditional practice, perhaps try making something else your meditation first, or exploring breath work and yoga if you are curious. These steps may, over time, open doors for you to explore meditation as and when you are ready, or perhaps they will serve you well enough that you won't need anything more. Either way, what have you got to lose?

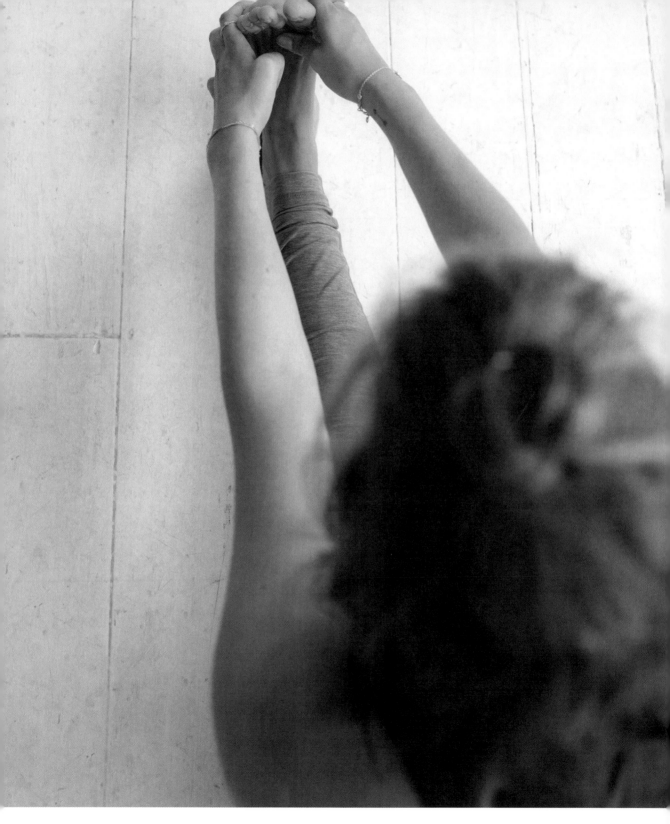

Exercise

Exercise can be amazing for the mind. For me, things like running become a form of meditation in themselves. The impact of exercise on the stress levels is so valuable in modern-day life, where chronic lack of time and endless pressures mean that lots of people experience unnatural amounts of stress on a daily basis.

Not only can we use physical activity as a means to distract ourselves when our minds are feeling busy, but there are also all sorts of chemical reactions that occur in the body when we exercise which make us feel good.

Therefore, it can be an incredibly useful way of relieving tension and keeping ourselves fit and healthy.

I'll come to talk about this more in the next chapter, but the most important thing is to decide which type of exercise works for you – find what you enjoy and what makes you feel good, as it is that which will do the most good for your mind as well as your body. Just as with any of these tools, pick what works, leave what doesn't and develop your own style of management to help you connect with and understand yourself.

Mind Round-up

There is no single big secret to finding happiness, so I would encourage you to let go of that concept. There is no master key that opens every single person's door to a balanced life and a healthy body and mind. So the bad news is that it can take a lot of work, of listening to yourself, trial and error, good and bad days, three steps forwards, two steps back … but the good news is that the key is there, it already exists and your challenge is to discover it within yourself. To me, that is a pretty exciting prospect and one that I hope you will be willing to explore with me.

One thing that is true for us all is that, without acceptance, we make it all a lot harder for ourselves. Striving for better is all well and good, but accepting the present situation for whatever it is will allow you to move forward. Really, it isn't about bettering yourself but more about understanding that you are already good enough. We live in a world of so much self-doubt and self-deprecation that it almost seems socially inappropriate to embrace ourselves for who we are; the idea of self-love can seem a wishy-washy hippie concept. If we can shift away from that fear of judgement and learn to love and accept ourselves, as well as others, we enable ourselves to get the most from life. So rather than focusing on bettering yourself, perhaps it is bettering the connection with yourself that will help you to create a more wholesome, happy and fulfilling life.

If you can learn a little more about how your mind works, you can establish a deeper relationship with yourself on an emotional level whereby you are more accepting and understanding of your own thoughts, feelings, emotions and actions. This allows you to choose the situations you place yourself in, meaning that you can start to cultivate relationships and environments that suit your wants and needs.

As you begin to recognize certain things about yourself, it is important to hold no judgement or expectation. Accepting who you are nurtures you in the most constructive and positive way. No matter how little time you may feel you have, creating space for this connection with yourself serves as an opening to a more positive internal environment. If you think in terms of attracting what you project, then this will inevitably affect so many other aspects of your life, weaving its way through how you think about yourself, others and the world around you.

Body

02

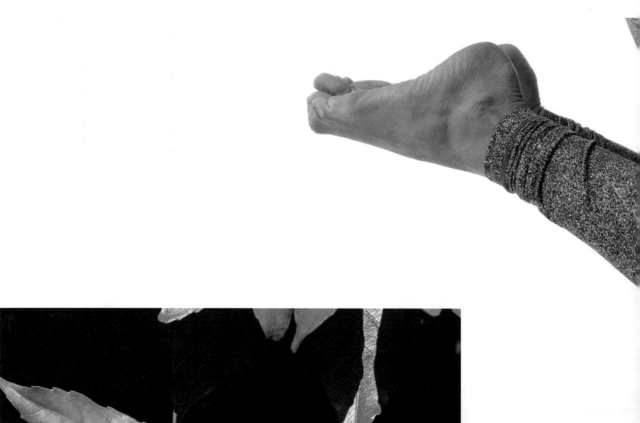

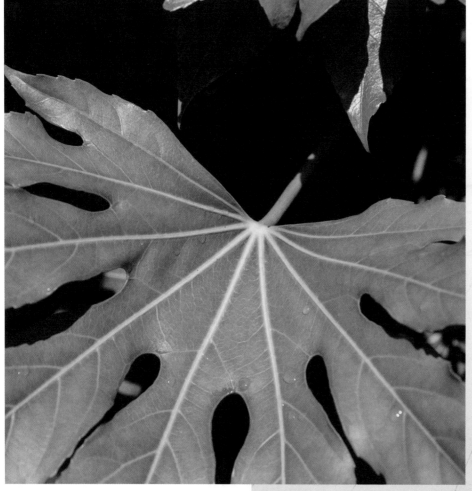

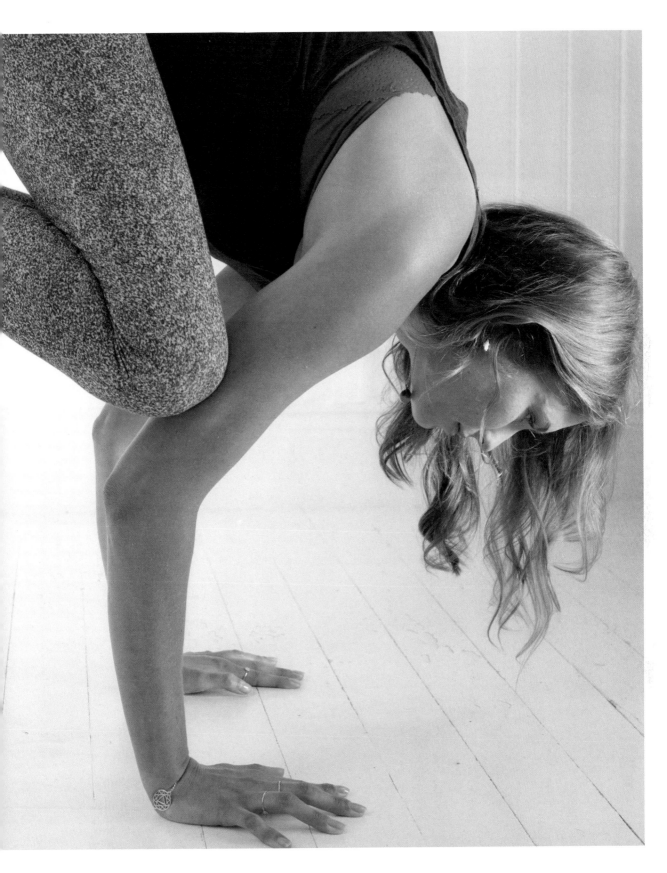

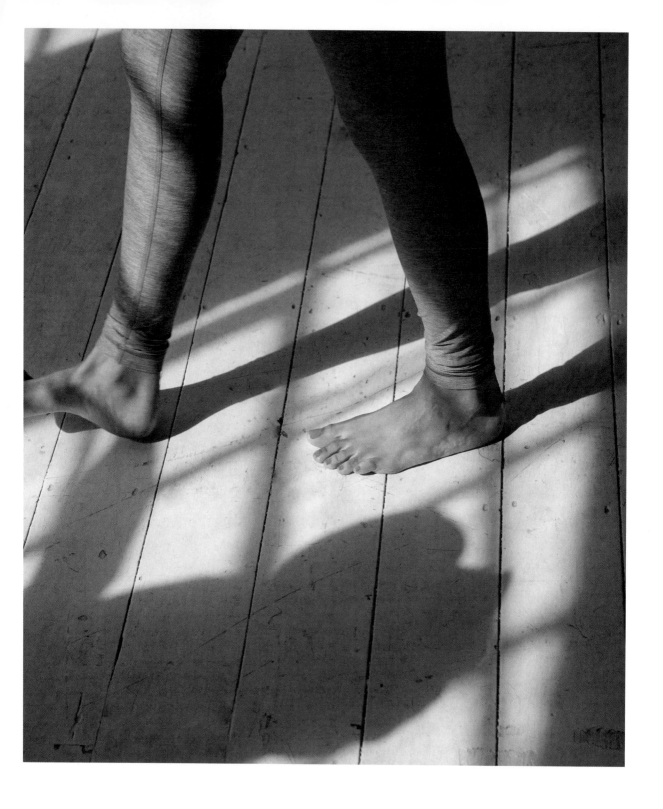

Every second, each cell in your body is working away without conscious instruction to provide you with all the vital functions needed in order to survive.

Every second, each cell in your body is working away without conscious instruction to provide you with all the vital functions needed in order to survive. In fact, many of the things that your body does are taken for granted most of the time. Often it isn't until we get injured, lose the ability to do something or find ourselves in a threatening situation that we even acknowledge certain functions of our bodies at all. Yet despite all the amazing things that our bodies do, many of us spend our lives being unduly harsh about them in one way or another. When we take the time to reflect on how we feel about and treat our bodies, we can begin to develop a much more positive relationship with them. Rather than criticize them, we should pursue and embrace a caring and loving attitude. By adopting this approach, the motivation to take care of yourself may come much more easily.

Practising Self-acceptance

A lot of people think about their bodies primarily from an aesthetic point of view, and as a result many have a difficult relationship with their physical self. It is so easy to make comparisons to others, especially via social media. It used to be that people compared themselves to celebrities and models in magazines, but now you can compare yourself to millions of people all over the world. It can be incredibly challenging to find peace with your own body when there is so much out there to make you feel inadequate. The truth is that we are all human and everyone faces different insecurities. The minute you learn to let go of these unfavourable comparisons, you create a more positive attitude towards yourself.

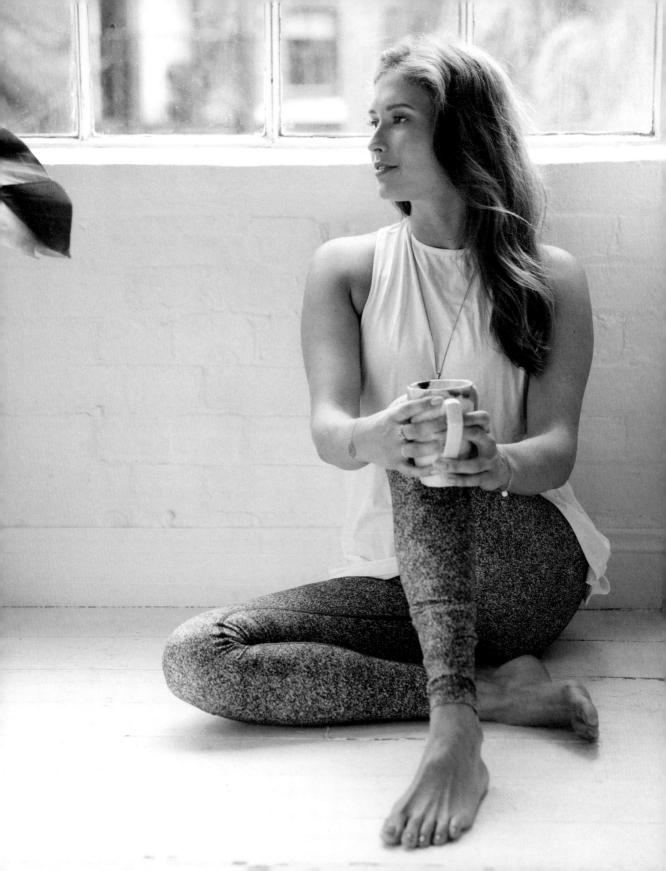

'What really matters is not the way you look, but the way that you feel, because that feeds into so many other aspects of your life.'

Feeling comfortable in your own skin can do so much to project confidence in other areas of your life, and that does not have to mean spending days on end pushing yourself through gruelling workouts to get your dream physique. It really starts with finding self-acceptance and applying that to the way you feel about your body. Most of us, I'm sure, have had moments when we are critical or upset about the way we look, and we are always much more critical towards ourselves than we would ever be to others. What really matters is not the way you look, but the way you feel.

Of course, that is easy to say – when you have things that you don't love about yourself, it is much easier to focus on them than on the bits that you do actually like. And aside from what you love or hate, how easy is it to forget what your body actually does for you? Every second of every day your body is doing thousands of things to keep you alive – so, regardless of how you feel about it from an aesthetic perspective, it is important to celebrate everything it does for you each day. Of course, for lots of us, the way we look can help us to feel more confident and that does serve a purpose in itself, but by shifting your mindset away from being critical, you can begin to accept that the body you have today is the one that will carry you around and that allows you to do so many things.

Sure – you might not have the abs you want, or you might have aches and pains that prevent you from feeling your best, but you only have this one body – so the best thing we can do is to accept it, look after it, protect it and love it. Of course, keeping yourself fit and healthy is important – not for aesthetic reasons but to make sure that you have the best chance of living a long, happy life with minimal discomfort and maximum enjoyment. So while you work towards any aesthetic goals, you can also try to focus some of your energy on accepting the way you look and feel, today. An important part of the journey is treating your body with respect so that it keeps working well in years to come.

No matter how much effort you put in every day to your work, fitness, friends, family and anything else, if you feed yourself negativity it is counter-productive to achieving your goals. No matter what happens today, know that you are where you are supposed to be. If you can find contentment in who and where you are right now, that positivity will flow through so many aspects of your life.

Rather than feeling insignificant compared to someone else, try to draw inspiration from what they are achieving and strive to be the best version of yourself. After all, you will always do 'you' better than anyone else can. With this shift in mindset, you will equip yourself to achieve great things. Set your own goalposts and create a mental environment where happiness comes first. *The Happiness Advantage* by Shawn Achor is a brilliant book which suggests that if we put our happiness first, we are more likely to achieve and exceed our goals. It makes total sense to me. If we wait to achieve something in the hope that it will bring happiness, by the time we achieve it the goalposts will have moved and we will never be content. Instead, we can try to enjoy the journey rather than focus on the destination, and apply that to every part of our lives if we can. If there are things we wish to change about ourselves, that is our prerogative, but if we can do it through love and nurturing rather than discontent, it brings a much more positive perspective to the situation and we're much more likely to find contentment.

The Importance of Exercise

There are many things that you can do to protect and nurture your body and keep it strong, healthy and functioning well. One of the most obvious is exercise. Many people spend a great proportion of their day sitting at desks due to the nature of their jobs. For those with more active jobs this is perhaps a little less of a concern – if you spend your time running around, or walking between appointments or meetings, then when you can't make it to the gym you know that you've at least had some movement throughout the day.

I really used to underestimate the effect of exercise on my mind as well as my body. I touched on it in the last section, but for me

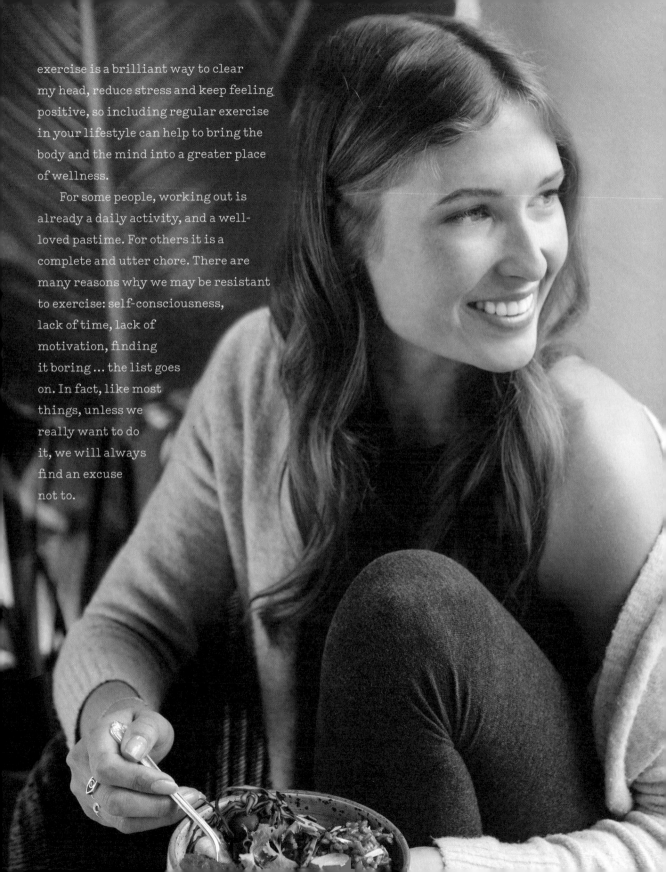

exercise is a brilliant way to clear
my head, reduce stress and keep feeling
positive, so including regular exercise
in your lifestyle can help to bring the
body and the mind into a greater place
of wellness.

For some people, working out is
already a daily activity, and a well-
loved pastime. For others it is a
complete and utter chore. There are
many reasons why we may be resistant
to exercise: self-consciousness,
lack of time, lack of
motivation, finding
it boring ... the list goes
on. In fact, like most
things, unless we
really want to do
it, we will always
find an excuse
not to.

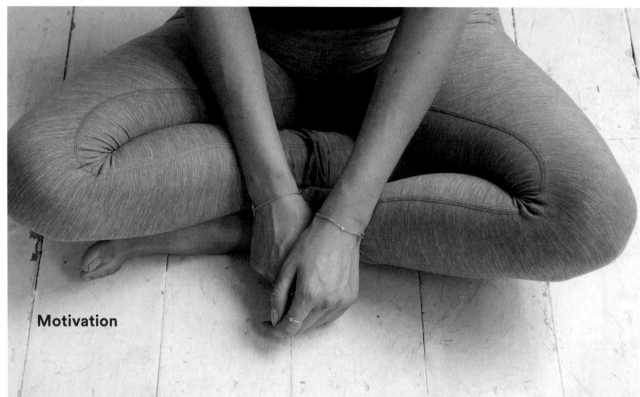

Motivation

For many people, the hardest part of exercise is getting started. If you are not particularly active and haven't paid much attention to keeping fit, the idea of stepping into a public gym or joining a group fitness class can be incredibly daunting. Going for a run can feel torturous, and powering through your thirty-minute cross-train at the gym is uninspiring if you can think of a hundred other things you would rather be doing. Injuries, long working hours and other commitments can leave exercise feeling like the lowest priority. This is really where the theory that one size doesn't fit all becomes apparent. The best trick, and you'll see a pattern emerging here, is to figure out what works for you.

You need to find the motivation not only to start something but also to keep it up, as consistency makes the process a lot easier. The easiest way to commit to exercise is to find a way to get moving that you actually enjoy – it doesn't have to be horrible, or boring. Of course, it might be tough to begin with as you build your fitness levels, but if you want to give yourself the best chance of keeping it up, explore lots of different types of sport and exercise to find the one that inspires you. I go through real phases and love to mix it up, but there is a lot to be said for consistency. I find balancing variety with committing to regular classes is a great way to notice changes in my body, as well as reap the benefits mentally. It really is so important to find something you enjoy – if you really hate running, then don't force yourself to run three times a week. You may also find that variety is beneficial when it comes to developing your fitness. However, you may find that a routine helps you commit to regular exercise. You can combine the two and enjoy different activities on different days, allowing yourself to mix things up but committing to each of them in a way that gives you structure (if that is how your mind and body work).

Having a workout buddy or booking yourself into a class is a great way to help you commit to exercising. The accountability of it, feeling like you're letting someone down or wasting money by not showing up, is sometimes the extra push we need. That said, remember you're doing it for you, and while you don't want to stand up a friend for that 6.30 a.m. spin class every week, it is OK to listen to your body properly and duck out on the days when you really need the rest, because that is just as important.

The price tag attached to gym memberships or classes can be totally off-putting and sometimes completely unaffordable. I've gone through various periods in my life where I've had higher or lower levels of disposable income and have had to alter my exercise schedule accordingly. There are so many free ways to work out now, or guides and plans available for a one-time fee, allowing you to work out at home. For lots of people this adds a level of ease and flexibility that is incredibly helpful in terms of fitting exercise around other commitments.

My biggest tip, which applies to any lifestyle change, would be to make working out as easy as possible. The fewer excuses you are able to make, the more likely you are to do it. If it is boring, switch it up. If you are lacking in motivation, find a friend to help drag you to the gym, or really take the time to think about why you want to do it. If it doesn't seem like a financial possibility, try to look into ways you can get moving without spending money. Help yourself to minimize excuses and hopefully you might even discover something you enjoy!

No matter how busy your life is, there are always ways to add movement to your days or weeks. Love a lazy weekend? Make time to keep fit in the week instead. Is there a shower at work? How about running or cycling there? Or running home (or even part of the way home)? These things sound simple, and they are – they just require a little forethought and experimentation. Also, be realistic – don't overcommit and set yourself up to fall short. That is a big demotivator.

The idea of fitting in a workout or finding time to prepare good food might seem totally ridiculous if it already feels as though there aren't enough hours in the day.

In my experience I find that the days and weeks where I squeeze in even the shortest of workouts and ensure that I eat fuelling food are when I am most productive. Exercising gives me a much clearer head, allowing me to focus better for the rest of the day. I usually like to work out first thing in the morning as it really invigorates me. It also ensures that exercise isn't the thing that gets dropped off the list when I run out of time to get everything done in the day. That said, when I know that I'm spending a day working from home, I quite like exercising later in the day in order to break things up a little. It's all about finding what works for you, but a great tip to try is scheduling whatever movement you choose into your day in advance and treating it like an important meeting, so that you really make it happen. It's a formula that I figured out over time, but now I know what I like, what makes me feel good and what I have time for, it makes it much easier to make movement a priority.

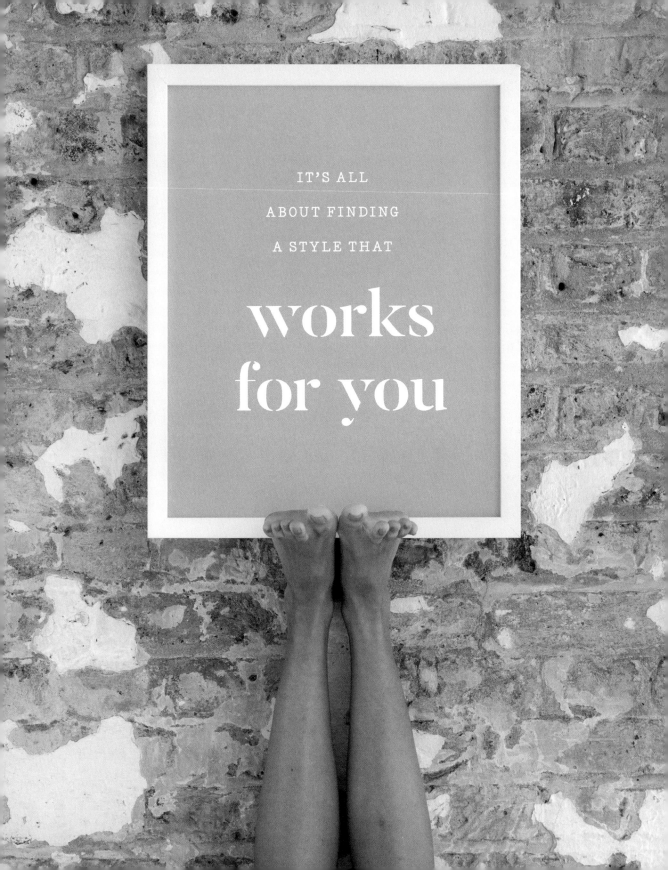

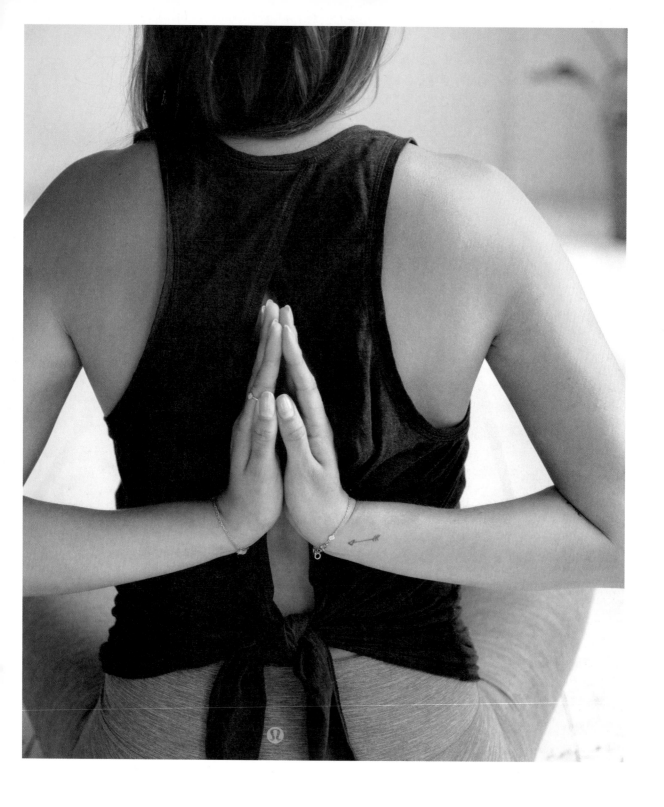

Yoga: Linking the Mind and Body

While writing this book I've really struggled over whether to talk about yoga in the Mind or the Body section, because it really draws the two together and shouldn't be categorized as one over the other. I will explain why.

I think my first encounter with yoga was when we were offered after-school sessions in the drama hall as a teenager. I don't remember very much, except that I was one of the few students who went to the class and on at least one occasion I fell asleep in savasana, much to the amusement of my friends. As a university student I joined my local Bikram yoga studio in the holidays and tried to complete thirty-day challenges, approaching it with a totally different mentality to how I think of yoga today. My focus was solely on the physical benefits, during a period of my life which involved long hours at the gym, desperately seeking fitness and a flat stomach. I hadn't

yet discovered how powerful yoga is for the mind, but I suppose it was a valuable part of my introduction to the practice.

Bikram was fast-paced, hard work and incredibly sweaty – much more familiar to me at the time in terms of a workout. I was totally unversed in sitting still or switching off the mind, so when I did try other styles of classes they seemed too slow and I thought they were a bit of a waste of time. My mind would wander in a class, embarrassed by my lack of flexibility, and I would ask myself why I didn't just stay behind to stretch a bit more after the gym? Little did I know that I was just a few short years away from not only practising yoga and meditation but actually loving them so much that I would be teaching them, too.

Having approached yoga from such a physical viewpoint, I never expected it to open so many doors on a deeper level. It is very easy to think of yoga as a form of exercise, a relaxation technique or a series of postures linked together, but really, true yoga goes so far beyond the physical asana practice. In fact, the physical asanas (postures) form just one of the limbs of yoga, a small part of something much greater. In the Western world we have begun to focus quite heavily on that physical aspect, but yoga is a whole lot more than that. The way you learn to face challenges during the practice can be applied to how you deal with problems you face elsewhere. You build confidence in your strength, which can then manifest itself in your self-confidence off the mat. Over time, it can really help you to understand who you are and connect you to your true self.

The most common thing I hear when people ask me about yoga is, 'But I can't even touch my toes!' This is exactly where they miss the whole point of yoga, by addressing it from a very physical point of view. Perhaps you want to use it as a form of exercise or to help you stretch out after a week at a desk, and those are great reasons to start practising yoga. But that is the point: you have to start somewhere and it is always an evolving practice, one that goes far beyond whether or not you can touch your toes.

Flexibility can be a real challenge when it comes to yoga. I used to be really embarrassed about my poor flexibility; I was quite strong when I first started, but those hours of building my strength and not stretching enough meant that I was nowhere near as supple as I would have liked. In fact, one of the reasons I really decided to give yoga a go was to help me recover from training at the gym. It can take quite a lot of mental strength to release your ego or self-consciousness and just accept the level you are at and work within the limitations of your own body. What I didn't realize was that strength was actually a very valuable asset to start with. It is quite easy for a flexible person to push further into a posture, relying on their flexibility to bend them into the pose. However, they may not necessarily be engaging the muscles that the

'Through a balance of strength and flexibility you can develop a powerful yoga practice.'

asana aims to activate. Having a base level of strength gives you a greater level of control within your practice.

Of course, that is not to say that one is more valuable than the other, and it certainly does not mean that you need either one in order to start yoga; it just shows that through a balance of strength and flexibility you can develop a strong practice. Everything will come with time and patience – the more you do, the stronger and suppler you will become. It can take months or years to get to grips with certain postures, and some people find it a lot more challenging than others. The key is to keep at it, to not compare yourself to anyone else, and to ask lots of questions.

If you feel as if you have been working towards something for a long time and it is still not clicking, talk to your teachers – the chances are you won't be the only one and they may be able to offer you hints and tips to help you take the next steps.

Yoga really is for everyone. There are so many different teachers, styles and postures that I am yet to meet a student who hasn't benefited from regular practice or found a class or teacher that really resonates with them. However, yoga doesn't have to be rigid and you really don't need to take it too seriously. If your local studio seems intimidating (or perhaps you don't have access to one at all), you can incorporate yoga into your other physical activities or at home. It is all about being mindful of the breath, and of course getting a good stretch, too.

Our bodies store not only physical tension, but also tension that builds up as a result of emotional experiences which we subconsciously hold on to. There are lots of different thoughts and theories about the connection between the mind and body, and at first I found it difficult to get my head around the concept that such a link existed.

The emotional impact of yoga I have seen on people has been incredibly moving, driving me to learn more about the mind–body connection and the way we store and hold on to tension.

I remember when I first felt emotional in a yoga class; I was really embarrassed about it. It happened a few times over the years, but I never gave it too much thought. Then while I was doing my training I was sent for a deep-tissue therapy massage to try to address a recurring injury in my neck and shoulder. The massage was incredibly strong and uncomfortable but I instantly noticed a reduction in the pain I had been experiencing.

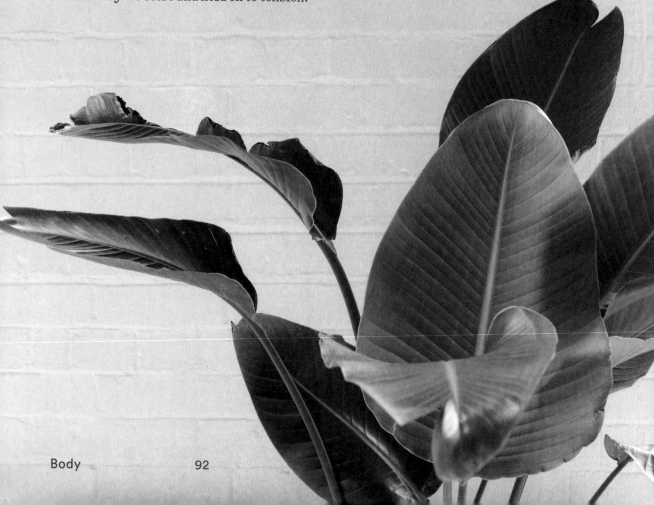

The next morning I arrived at the shala to do our morning practice and within minutes I was in floods of tears. At first I tried to hold them back, but then I realized that the release was important. I cried continuously for the full ninety minutes of my practice, and walked out of the shala feeling like a whole new person. Totally out of nowhere I had been overwhelmed by emotion despite not feeling as though anything was wrong at all. Where the massage therapist had worked into my tension, he had worked out more than the physical and I was experiencing an emotional response as a result.

We hold so much stress in our bodies and it can build up, causing discomfort or even pain. Yoga helps to connect the mind and body, allowing you to release this tension and to free you from the stresses you are holding onto.

I have now seen this time and time again with myself as well as with my students when we work on a specific area of the body, resulting in a much deeper release. This can lead to feelings of deep emotion or even cause us to cry. The unfamiliarity of this can be a little disconcerting the first few times it happens, but if you are feeling teary during or after class, it is totally normal and the best thing you can do is embrace it to allow the body to let go of what it has been holding onto. Yoga postures can largely be grouped together, and there are two main asana groups which are commonly related to this sort of emotional release – chest- or heart-openers (or back bends) and hip-openers – which I will talk about in a little bit.

The funny thing is that sometimes you might not even realize that you are holding onto anything. For some people there are obvious traumas that of course they can't help but be aware of, but for others it may be something they can't even remember – an emotion repressed over time, however great or insignificant. The most important thing is not to judge it too much or try to understand why. Just allow it to happen and ride whatever comes up in your practice.

So Where to Start?

Well, as mentioned, the breath is a great place to begin, and the exercises in the last chapter will help you – but I appreciate that you may want to approach yoga from a more physical place. I would encourage everyone to begin yoga under the guidance of a qualified teacher, purely to help you build solid foundations upon which to develop your practice. Many studios offer beginners' courses where you can learn the basics over a series of weeks, or even weekly classes that you can dip into when it suits you.

It can be incredibly daunting when you start to learn something new. For lots of people the idea of stepping into a room and exposing our physical weaknesses is pretty scary, especially if we have a competitive nature. I'll give you one piece of reassurance here: no one will be looking at you. I don't mean that in a negative way, but the only people who might be looking around the room are the ones who are just as unsure as you are. There is nothing to be self-conscious about and every person in that room is or was a beginner at some point. It is easier said than done, but if you can step out of your comfort zone, you will open the door to so many wonderful things.

If, for whatever reason, you cannot get to classes, there are many online resources that make it easy to start yoga in the comfort of your own home (and this applies to exercises, too). The internet gives you access to lots of subscription services where you can browse hundreds of yoga videos, which vary from ten-minute flows to a ninety-minute class, so you can always fit it around your busy life. You can also use resources such as YouTube to access videos for free without committing to a subscription plan. I would offer a few pieces of advice if you choose to follow yoga tutorials online or on DVD:

Always make sure that the video has been made by a qualified yoga teacher. Social media in particular has given rise to so many people offering advice without qualifications, and while they may provide a valuable resource and a lot of inspiration, be mindful of yourself and the way in which you are moving your body. The same goes for nutrition, exercise and lots of other things. I would be wary of following guidance from certain sources without seeking professional advice.

Try to listen to the cues more than you watch. By looking up at the screen you may be compromising your alignment and the last thing you want is to injure yourself.

Remember that your body is likely to be very different from that of the person on screen. There are such huge variations between our anatomies, so forcing yourself into postures to look like something that you have seen someone else do is probably not going to be good for your body. This is where working with a teacher to understand the foundations can be really beneficial, but if you are going it alone, just be very mindful of individual differences and personal limitations.

Start slowly. It can be so tempting to rush into trying lots of fun things like inversions or deep back bends, but just be mindful again of your body and ensure that you are both warm and physically able to safely try whatever you are doing without direct instruction. Have fun, but keep your body safe, as you've only got the one to live with!

Body

Some Basic Yoga Postures

I thought a lot about including some yoga routines in this book, but for the reasons mentioned I haven't felt totally comfortable with providing words and pictures to guide you through a practice. I came instead to the conclusion that a way of sharing some of my teaching would be to offer a little bit of understanding about how the practice of yoga can help with some common issues in the body. In the following pages you will find descriptions of a few groups or types of postures which you will come across in classes, books and online – or you can watch my videos on my website and on YouTube – to help you to understand the reasons why they are practised. Each group of asanas has specific benefits aimed at improving physical and emotional health and well-being.

You'll find lots of detailed instructions about how to safely practise yoga on the Mind Body Bowl YouTube channel.

Twists

In a twist, space is created in between the vertebrae, lengthening the spine and stretching the back muscles. This helps to develop and maintain a good range of motion in the spine, and creates space for energy to flow more freely, making twists an instantly energizing asana group.

In addition to what they do for your spine, twists are also brilliant for aiding digestion. They help to stimulate the organs which can improve the function of the digestive system, so try them if you're feeling bloated or sluggish. For those of you who struggle with digestive issues, or maybe are just having a bit of an off day, twists and forward folds in yoga can be a great way to relieve digestive discomfort.

A really simple exercise that you can do which may help to relieve stomach ache or trapped wind is a gentle lying-down twist. It is really important to listen to your own body and try this only if you feel comfortable in doing so. This works well for me, but it is worth discussing it with someone who knows your medical history if you are unsure of whether or not to try it.

Lie down flat with both shoulders on the ground. Keeping the left leg extended, draw the right knee into the chest, hugging it there for a few breaths. Then, using the left hand, draw the right knee across the body, extending the right arm out to the side and gazing towards the right fingertips. Keep working the right knee down to the left side while the right shoulder grounds down into the mat. Stay here for as long as you like, then inhale to come back to centre and repeat on the other side.

It is worth noting that it is recommended that you engage the core muscles to protect and support the spine when you are twisting. An inhalation is also used to lengthen the spine, and an exhalation to twist, ensuring that you first create space, before rotating.

Back Bends/Heart-openers

Back bends, otherwise known as heart-openers, are a really valuable group of asanas from both a physical and emotional perspective. They are a fundamental part of many yoga sequences and their many benefits include strengthening and aligning the spine. Lots of us spend a large part of our days folded or hunched forwards, such as while working at a desk or computer, and so it's good to counteract this repetitive action and help us to realign the spine.

As you bend the back you also open up the chest, releasing muscular tension and creating openness around the heart and lungs, allowing us the space to breathe more deeply. It is not unusual to feel emotional after completing heart-openers, and in fact I find that they can help to relieve a build-up of anxiety and emotion as a result of this physical release.

In order to deepen a back bend, you need to create length at the front of your body. Stretching the hip flexors, for example, can create additional mobility, which allows you to work into a stronger back-bending practice.

You don't have to engage in extreme back bends to benefit from them – gentle postures can still have a significant effect on the body and are a really great way to prepare for more powerful back bends as your yoga practice develops.

Back bends can be quite scary, but as you learn to trust yourself and overcome self-imposed limits and expectations, you will develop a strength of mind that can be applied to other areas of your life.

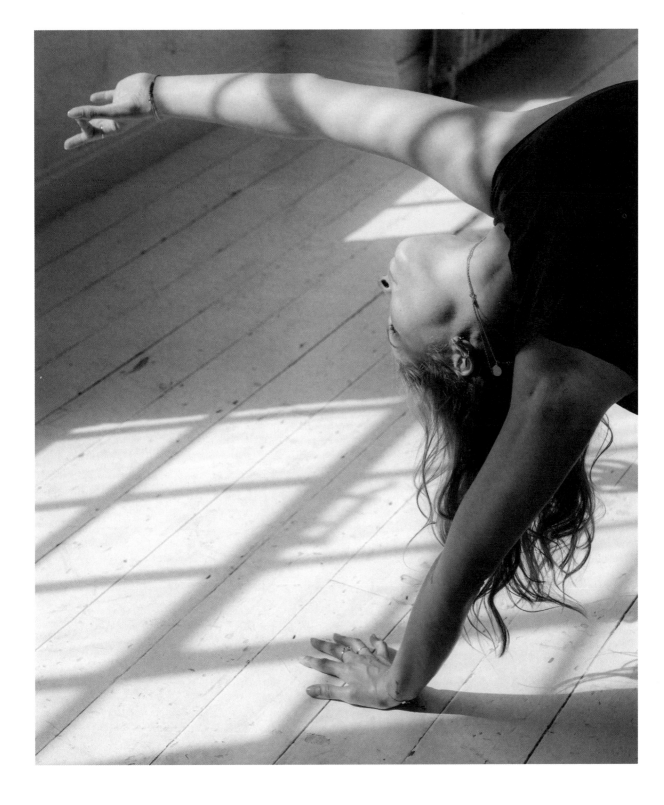

Body

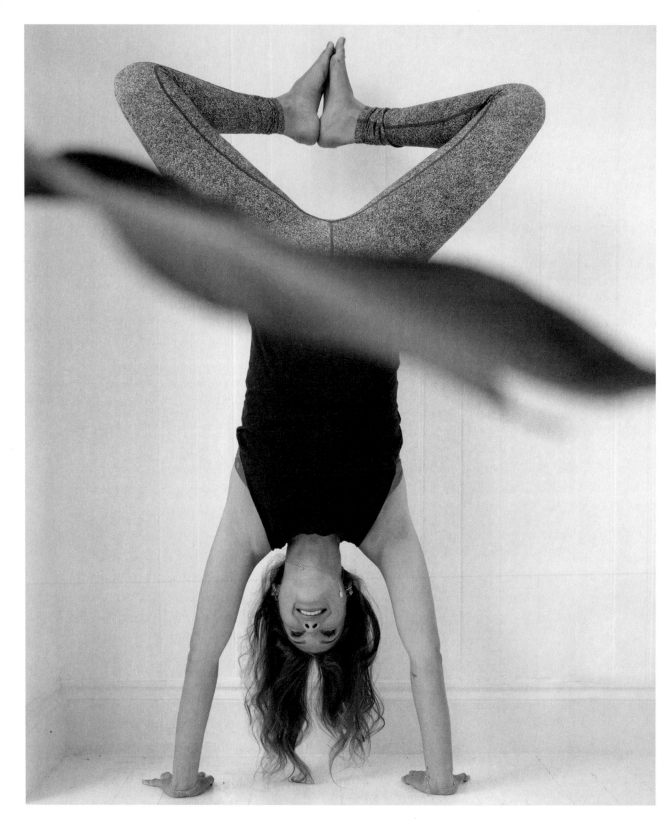

Hip-openers

Many of us have tight hips as a result of spending long periods of time sitting down. Not only can tight hips be felt in themselves, but for some people this can have repercussions on other parts of the body, such as the pelvis and lower back. Through hip-openers you can work on the muscles and joints in and around the hips, and prevent tension and strain in the area.

You may find that the effect is fairly instantaneous and you may notice increased mobility in the hip joint almost immediately. Hip-openers can offer emotional as well as physical benefits, serving to relieve those suffering from stress and anxiety by releasing emotion stored in this part of the body.

Hip-openers can be really strong so, as with all postures, be mindful not to go too deep too quickly. Allow your body time to open up and adjust, both in each individual practice, and over time in general.

Inversions

If you use social media platforms such as Instagram, you may think that to be a true yogi you have to master all the different hand-stands, head-stands and other crazy tricks you see all over your feed. You absolutely do not! But as well as being incredibly addictive once you start to learn them, inversions are actually really good for you.

Generally speaking, an inversion is any posture where your heart is above your head, so that gravity is sending blood to the brain. This makes inversions wonderfully energizing and invigorating on a physical and mental level. More gentle inversions are relaxing – a simple half-shoulder stand, for example – and can be used to calm the nervous system and bring balance to the body.

Inversion practice is fun, and there is a lot to be said for releasing your inner child and not taking yoga, or yourself, too seriously! It can also build confidence. Of course, like anything, be careful to protect your body and maintain a safe practice.

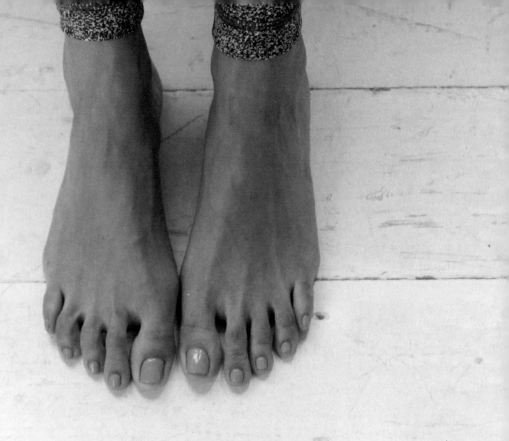

Getting the Foundations Right

It can be pretty exciting when you start to notice your progress in a new challenge, and yoga is no exception to that. No matter how much I try to tell myself that my asana practice is not about how many poses I can do, I still feel a sense of achievement when I crack something properly for the first time. It can be tempting to jump ahead and try advanced postures because they look fun or would make a great party trick or Instagram picture. I can't stress enough the importance of taking time to build a strong foundation in your practice before trying anything advanced. Not only will this keep you safe but it will also mean that when you do start to progress your practice, you will probably do so more quickly because you will have built up the necessary strength.

As with any exercise, it is really important to warm up properly and ease into deeper postures, such as hip-openers and back bends. This will help to keep your body safe and reap the most benefit from your practice.

Limitations

We all have physical and mental limitations in life, and yoga is no exception. In my own experience the two are often linked: I associate things I find physically challenging with negative thought patterns.

Here is an example: I have always found some deep back-bending postures quite challenging. The tightness in my hip flexors meant that I found it difficult to really get anywhere with the poses. I was also incredibly tight across the chest and shoulders, and my physical challenges translated into a sense of anxiety towards certain postures. As time went on I began to build up a real resistance to certain postures during class.

Eventually I decided I needed to overcome my fear of one particular pose (known as 'full wheel'). As my practice developed, the muscles at the front of my body lengthened and I became stronger, allowing my back bend to deepen. A lot of tension was released from my shoulders and chest over time, so I was able to push into the pose with much greater ease.

However, due to the compression point in my shoulders, despite all the amazing progress I felt I was making with this particular posture, my hands were still no closer to being aligned under my shoulders and I kept trying to force them without any luck. Once I learned about the compression points, which are to do with the structure of our bones and joints and the way in which they meet – something we can't change – I realized that it was futile to keep trying to force my arms and, in fact, I could cause myself harm by doing so. I began to relax more into the posture, learning to accept and enjoy where I am each day.

There is no such thing as a perfect asana and individual physical differences have to be kept in mind. If your flexibility is preventing you from getting deeper into a posture, that is something you can work on over time. However, if it is your anatomy – for example, the compression point in a joint – that may be a limitation you are unable to change. Don't try to fit your body into the pose; adjust and modify the pose to suit your body.

Natural Beauty

Lots of us are becoming increasingly conscious about what we are putting into our bodies, but how many think about what goes on them as well? Not only can you do a lot to help your body physically, but if you really want to look after yourself you might also want to consider the products you use on your hair and skin.

It took me a year or so into my new lifestyle to realize that although I was incredibly conscious about the toxins in my food, I was still putting harmful products on my skin, and skin absorbs a lot of what we expose it to. A big part of a healthy lifestyle for some of us will include shifting towards more natural products with fewer nasty ingredients. It can

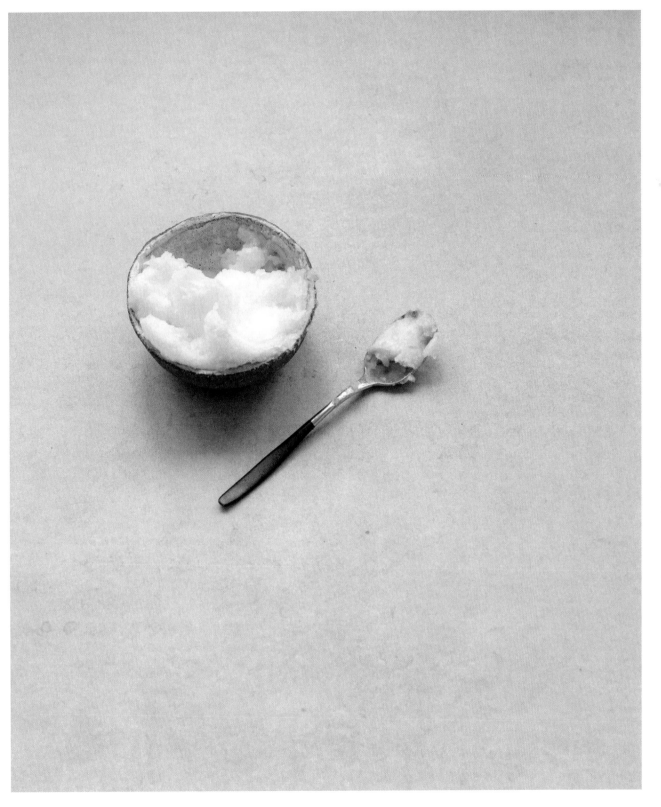

Body

'Lots of us are becoming more and more conscious about what we are putting in our bodies, but how many think about what goes on them as well?'

be pretty challenging to get your head around the names of ingredients and what you should and shouldn't worry about. For me, the easiest solution has been finding a few brands that I have come to know and trust, and generally sticking with them. I really enjoy hearing about and trying new products, but I soon realized that simplicity is pretty key (as with most things, really – you'll see how I apply that to food in the next section). Sticking to a small number of useful products is easier and more cost effective, and means you don't need to carry so much if you are going away. Experiment with natural products and find a routine that works for you. You don't have to spend a fortune – keep things modest and simple.

Hair care is a great place to start when it comes to cleaning up your bathroom act, especially for anyone who has caused damage through bleaching, straightening or whatever else you might have put it through. In my experience, combined with a healthy diet, using natural hair care can be a complete game-changer. I've tried everything from coconut oil masks to apple cider vinegar rinses, and religiously use a natural shampoo and conditioner, which have totally transformed my previously thin, brittle hair.

If you feel like taking things one step further, once a week or so you can try a coconut oil mask on your hair, which acts as a deep conditioning treatment. Leave it on overnight

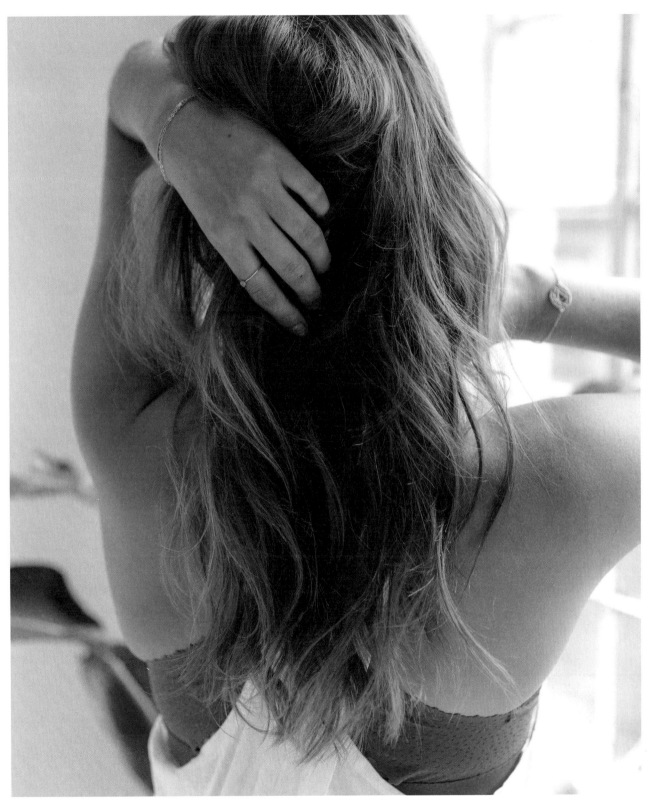

Body

'With one pot of coconut oil
you can almost totally transform
your wash bag.'

and then wash your hair as normal the next morning. If you have a build-up of product in your hair, try diluting apple cider vinegar in water (2–4 tablespoons vinegar in 500ml water) and rinsing with it before you get out of the shower, leaving it in your hair – I promise it doesn't smell once it dries! This helps to get rid of any residue of heavy products that might be making your hair feel limp or dull, and it really does work.

Another key swap is deodorant. There are so many natural alternatives to the chemical-filled products that we are used to. Again, it may take some experimenting, but for something we use every day, it really is the first thing I would encourage you to change in your beauty routine.

Depending on where you live, it may not be easy to get your hands on clean beauty products, and even if you do find them in a health store, it can still be incredibly difficult to decipher what is natural and what is actually just clever marketing. For that reason I try to strip things back as much as possible and even make my own products from ingredients that I have at home already. Coconut oil is an all-round saviour and is a great place to start. Some of its uses include (but are not limited to) the following:

01 moisturizer

02 make-up remover

03 teeth-whitener

04 hair mask/
conditioning treatment

05 after-sun (NOT
to be used before sun
exposure – you don't
want to fry your skin!)

With one pot of coconut oil you can almost totally transform your wash bag – not only saving yourself from nasty chemicals but also allowing you to travel much lighter, too.

As with changing any sort of beauty regime, if you choose to switch to more natural products there may be a transition period where your skin might not look or feel its best. A little trial and error is sometimes necessary to get your 'clean' skincare routine right and figure out what works for you.

Be kinder to the environment

Not only are natural beauty products kinder to your skin, hair and body in general, but they are also often gentler on the environment. The fewer harmful chemicals we all use, the less the impact on the world around us – so not only do we help ourselves, but we also help the environment.

You can extend this idea to other products in your home, such as what you use for cleaning. You will find it's not that difficult to minimize your impact on both people and nature by making your home as chemical-free as you can. There are some really great products on the market and if you can't pick them up in your local grocery store, have a browse online. They can be fairly competitive in price, if you are willing to shop around – and even if they are a little more expensive, I tend to find they last longer so are actually good value for money. If you are a fan of smelly candles or air fresheners, perhaps you might want to check the ingredients on those, too, as some of the commercial ones on the market are not necessarily made of things you want to be breathing in at home. It is so easy to make the transition to a more natural home environment, and I've found that as I've taken those steps in other areas of my life, it has become a natural process to bring these types of changes into my home, too.

Body Round-up

Lots of us are likely to experience some sort of dissatisfaction with our bodies at one point or another. Accepting this is, in itself, a big step, but we must make sure we nurture and respect our bodies, so that they can keep us active and able to do the things we love to do.

It is totally normal to want to work on certain parts of yourself, but try to find ways to love the skin you are in as much as possible, knowing that without it you wouldn't exist. Confidence is something that we can all wear if we just become more forgiving of ourselves. Look after yourself in a way that makes you feel good – find a way to stay active that you enjoy, and let go of comparisons if you find yourself holding onto them. You are not defined by the way you look, but if you want to work hard to change something so that you feel confident and happy, then that is amazing, too. Look after the one body you have and know that by feeling good about yourself, you will gain so much more than a healthy, happy appearance – that confidence really does filter through to other areas of your life and creates a happier, more loving environment.

Bowl

—03

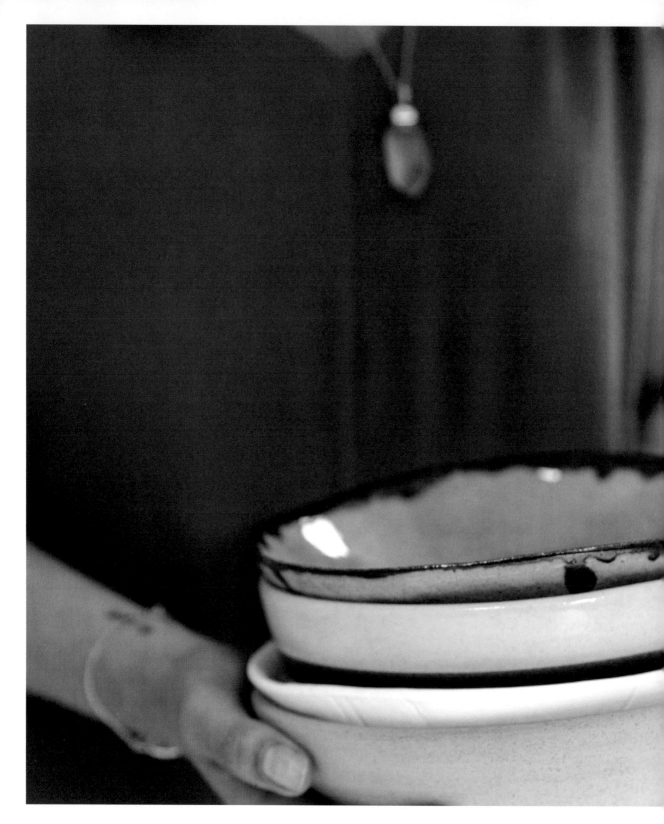

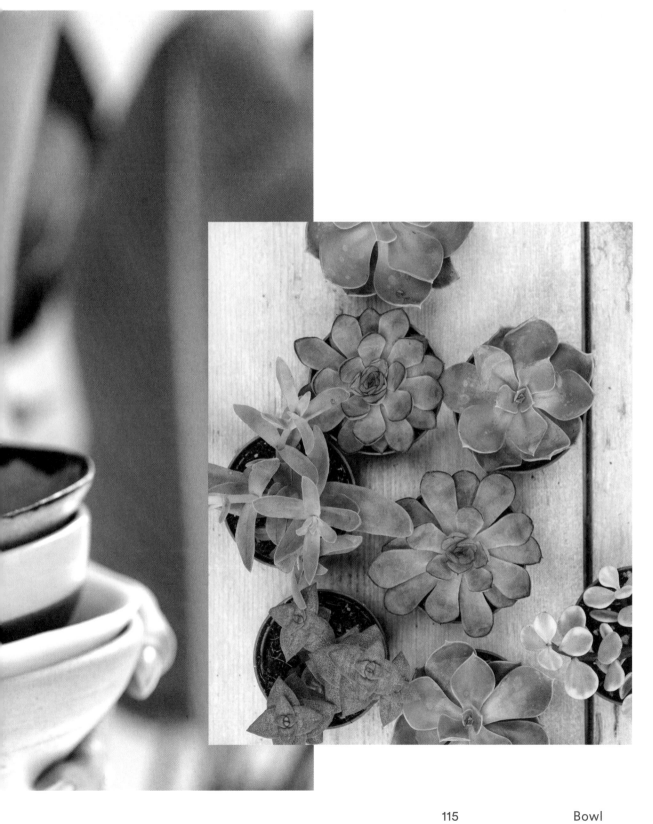

The more I have learned about and understood my body, the more I realize that you don't have to miss out on delicious food.

For some people food is sustenance, for others it is the root of social activity or a hobby that we enjoy indulging in. I think for lots of us there is something wonderful about food that goes far beyond taste. It is social, and our interest in and love of different foods brings people together all over the world.

I grew up in a family obsessed with food. My sister and I only came to realize this recently, but with two foodie parents their passion was bound to rub off on us at some point. I have memories of following delicious smells through the house into the kitchen and picking at whatever was cooking while no one was looking. We learned to cook fairly

early on, and many of our meals were freshly prepared from scratch at home (although cheesy pasta was a firm favourite for years, particularly when topped with a generous portion of tomato ketchup – much to my mum's disgust). But we also loved processed food and sugary treats, and my parents allowed us to eat them fairly freely. Food for me has always been so much more than fuel, and it therefore forms a crucial part of my personal idea of balance.

Some people can eat anything without it impacting the way they feel, but I and many others are incredibly sensitive to the food that we eat and it can dramatically affect our mental and physical well-being. In fact, adapting your diet to suit your body can be very enlightening. The more I have learned about and understood my body, the more I realize that you don't have to miss out on delicious food in order to be healthy.

We are all entitled to treat our bodies however we choose. Your decision to embark on a certain diet or regime shouldn't be criticized as long as it is done in a healthy, well-considered and informed way. The trouble is that you can find yourself committing to certain plans without fully understanding how your body may react and what it really needs. This can put you at risk of neglecting the fundamental nutritional requirements needed to maintain good health. Of course, my diet is restricted by the things that do and don't agree with my body, but I don't feel at all deprived because I fill my plate with a variety of delicious, fresh foods that taste good and leave me feeling good, too. I suppose the key is education – not necessarily what you learn from external sources, but a combination of understanding key principles and recognizing your own needs, habits and feelings.

Another concern I have with dieting is its association with 'success' or 'failure', being 'good' or 'bad', and the impact that might have on our view of ourselves. A specific diet plan can actually be a positive starting point for people who are confused about where to begin or who need a sense of structure to motivate themselves to commit to change. However, sustainable changes that suit your lifestyle and body are so much more valuable than short-term quick fixes. This is where the concept of acceptance ties back in. If you can learn to accept where you are in your life right now and move forward with a long-term attitude, you can look beyond a quick fix and actually create something more sustainable and positive.

If someone had said to me a few years ago that I needed to get in tune with my body, I would have looked at them with a blank face and thought they were talking nonsense – 'What on earth does that mean?'

'After all, we are constantly changing and what our bodies need from one day, week, month or year to the next can vary substantially.'

Well, now I am that person, here to advocate listening intently to your gut, your energy, to every sensation within you and using it as a guide for your actions, eating habits, social interaction and pretty much every aspect of your life.

In particular, one of the most important things that I have become aware of is my gut. Now I am much more conscious of how what I eat and do affects my digestive health. I have learned what different feelings in my body generally mean, and how I can best react to them. But this understanding has not come overnight and I am definitely still learning every day. After all, we are constantly changing and what our bodies need from one day, week, month or year to the next can vary substantially. If you want to work with the hints your body is giving you, the trick is to be adaptive and accepting.

Sometimes we can make changes to the sorts of foods we eat and feel amazing for it for a certain period of time. Then, without warning, the needs of our body change and we may no longer feel our best. At that point, we need to re-evaluate and adjust our diets accordingly.

Of course, this takes a good amount of trial and error, which can be frustrating at times, but experience helps you to be aware of your body's signals and signs, and you begin to understand how to cater to whatever it is you need.

It can be so hard to start recognizing what your body needs, but there are a few things you can ask yourself to help you tune in:

How do you feel? Don't just think in terms of 'good', 'bad', 'fine', etc.

What can you actually feel if you think about it?

Do you spend a lot of time with digestive discomfort, headaches, low energy? Are your bowel movements regular/irregular?

Are there certain things that trigger these feelings?

Or do they set in at certain times within the day?

Are there things that you habitually do in order to remedy these sensations?

Once you begin to listen to what your body is saying, you can start to respond to it. It may even be worth keeping a diary to track how you feel at certain times of the day; this will help you pinpoint the relationship between food, exercise, stress, other factors and the way you feel.

For your diet to be sustainable, it needs to fit into your lifestyle without too much fuss. The easier you make it for yourself, the much more likely you are to stick with it indefinitely, especially if and when you begin to notice a difference in the way it makes you feel.

Eating well is often associated with spending lots of money on expensive superfoods, but eating a diet beyond your financial means is not realistic or sustainable in the long run. In reality you don't need to spend hundreds of pounds on fancy ingredients. Of course, there is a market for these products and having them available is no bad thing if they appeal to certain people, but eating well doesn't have to be limited to those with lots of disposable income.

We all have different budgets when it comes to food shopping and we have to appreciate our financial limitations when it comes to any part of our lifestyle. The trick is to work within your means and find food that tastes good and gives you everything you need.

It is all too easy to think that spending a lot of money when you start a new regime is essential if you're going to enjoy what you're eating. I ended up with endless packets and jars of ingredients I would use once or twice before the 'best before' date and then have to throw out. Remember that good food is simple food, and eating well is about eating natural. It doesn't need to be fussy and you don't have to spend your time endlessly baking brownies just to use up the raw cacao powder that you needed in that energy ball recipe one time!

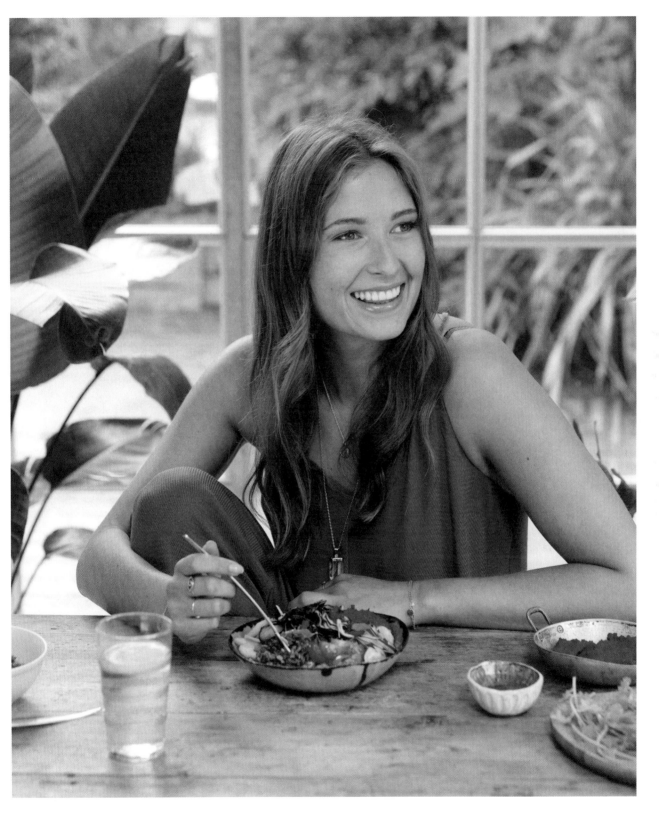

Bowl

Overcoming Common Hurdles

Breaking Bad Habits

Lots of us have bad habits when it comes to food. Skipping meals, grazing throughout the day and overeating are just some of the things that can be overcome if you take a more mindful approach to the way you eat. There are many reasons why you may eat mindlessly – for example, when you are distracted during meal times, perhaps trying to multi-task or talk to friends and family, you are not giving your full attention to eating. You therefore may not recognize how much you are eating and when you are full.

So many people I talk to say their biggest issue is the 4 p.m. slump, when they experience a sweet craving in order to get them through the rest of the afternoon. Over the years we have created this sugar roller-

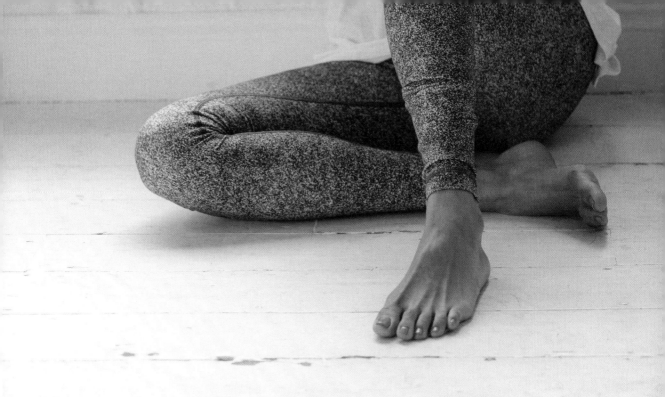

coaster where our blood sugar levels spike after eating refined sugar (not necessarily sweets – think sandwiches or even salads where the sugar is hidden away in dressings or bread) and then crash just an hour or so later. This crash will inevitably lead to more sugar cravings and then we are back on the roller-coaster again. For many people that is what 'normal' feels like and until they break the cycle, they don't recognize that they could feel so much better. With blood sugar levels peaking and troughing in such an extreme way, it can be impossible to ever feel fully energized. Another habit that you may have developed, and can perhaps consider breaking, is the association of certain activities with eating. For example, watching a film at the cinema or even at home can go hand in hand with filling up on a big bag of sweets or popcorn. Of course, from time to time there is something fun and comforting about curling up with snacks on the sofa, but if it happens too frequently it is a habit that you may choose to address to reduce your intake of processed, sugary foods.

Perhaps you always stop in for your favourite treat when you pass a particular shop, or maybe you get to certain times in the day and automatically reach for a snack without thinking whether or not you are actually hungry. While I completely advocate a liberal approach to the way you eat, being more mindful about your diet can really help to break these bad habits.

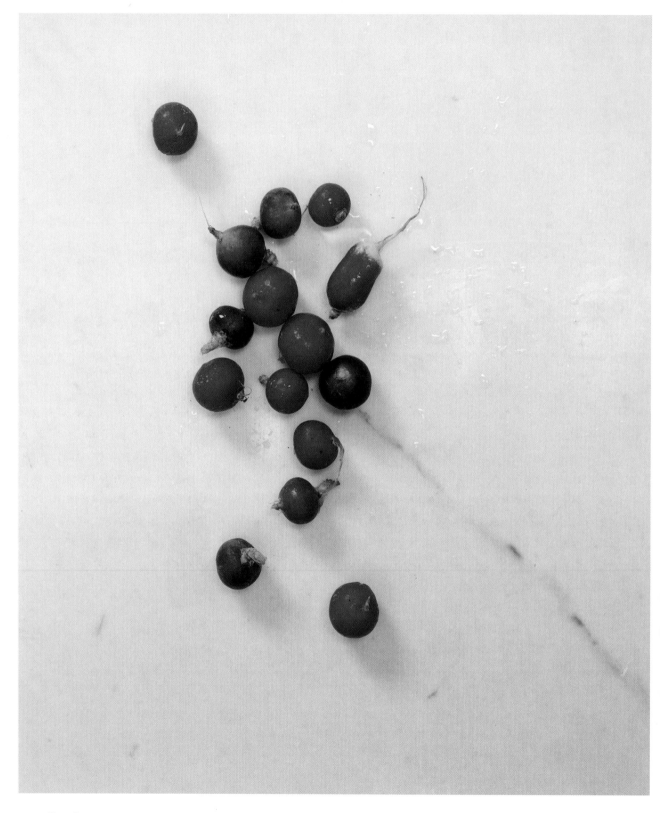

Flavour

When you first change your diet, one of the things you might struggle with is flavour. You may find that the new foods you are trying taste a little bland. Despite following other people's tried-and-tested recipes, I was a little disappointed with their lack of flavour. Even if you have always eaten a lot of fresh food, you may be used to including processed foods in your diet, too. These are typically higher in sugar and salt than something you might make at home. If you eat these processed foods regularly, your taste buds become suppressed and therefore less sensitive to subtle flavours. As a result you may feel you need to add more and more salt or sugar to your food in order to enhance its flavour and 'make it taste better'. Remember that by changing your diet and the ingredients you use, you can retrain your taste buds.

In as little as four weeks, you can start appreciating flavour differently – perhaps quite a bland time for a food lover – but in hindsight, it is a small price to pay. In my experience you can adapt your tastes fairly quickly. I now notice an abundance of flavour in the simplest foods, making cooking with, and eating, fresh, healthy food a lot more exciting. I can imagine that for some people the transition could take a little longer or be a little trickier, but I would urge you to stick with it long enough to allow yourself to adapt.

Eating Out

If you're trying to make healthy changes to your diet, eating out can be a little trickier. For the first few months, post diet-change, I became a bit anti-social and started missing out on quality time with friends and family. I knew this wasn't sustainable though, so took some steps to make sure that I could maintain my diet-change and still enjoy food with others. When invited to a friend's house for dinner, for example, I would discuss with them what they were planning to make. If they had planned something that I knew I couldn't eat, I asked if it would be OK to bring my own food, politely of course, as I didn't want to create extra work for them. When eating in a restaurant, I'd call ahead to find out more about the food they served. Lots of restaurants will happily create something simple for you.

I started to realize the importance of having confidence in your decisions. I chose to stick to the way of eating that suits my body all the time, and I did so because that is what makes me feel best. It has absolutely nothing to do with anyone else and so, in the sort of situation where you are ordering in a restaurant and can't spot something on the menu that works for you, be confident in asking for a little help.

Crucially, however, just because you want to make healthy changes doesn't mean you have to stick with them 100 per cent of the time. If you find that a more casual approach works best for you, then making small changes even some of the time will still make for amazing results. Remember not to over-commit and leave yourself open to feeling disappointed if you don't follow through every single time. Make it manageable and be kind to yourself.

Top tips for eating out:

If invited to a friend's for dinner, ask what they are planning to cook and offer to help or bring food if you think you will struggle. Planning ahead means less of a fuss at the dinner table and your host will hopefully be more understanding.

Call restaurants in advance – let them know your dietary preferences and discuss options so that you don't feel pressured when the waiter comes to take your order.

If in doubt or really stuck, most places will offer you simple veg – just be confident enough to ask.

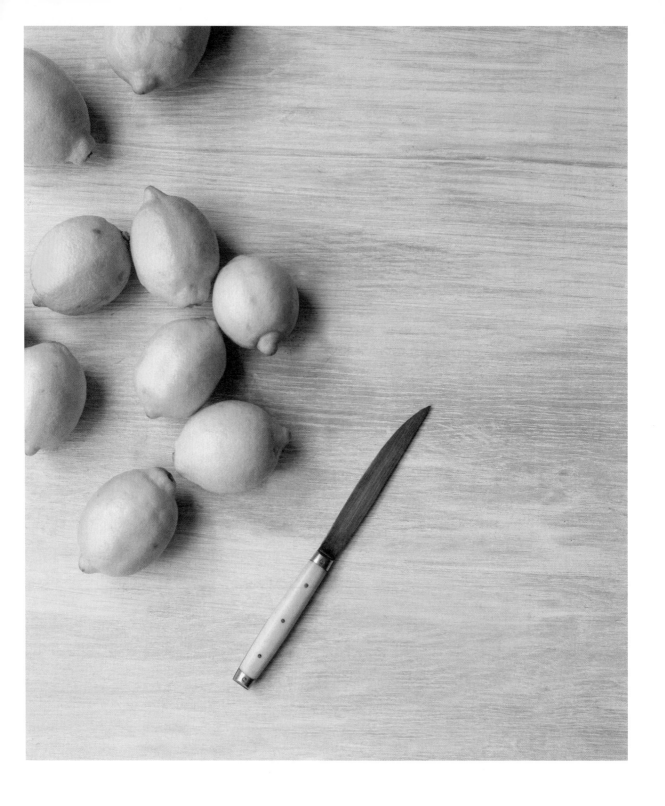

Bowl

Simplicity is key

For a lot of us, even if we love to cook, food is so often about convenience. The majority of our meals are likely to be based around whatever is going on during our working week, so finding simple foods that don't compromise on taste is really helpful. I have a few dishes that I know I can go to again and again, sometimes a few times a week when things are busy, knowing they can be prepared and eaten with minimal hassle, but still taste good and give me the energy that I need.

When I began collating recipe ideas for this book, I wanted to show the simplicity of the sort of food you can create with as little fuss as possible. I love to cook and when I'm throwing a dinner party I usually spend a day experimenting with more complicated ideas and trying to get a little more fancy, but that makes up such a tiny proportion of my cooking. Most days, cooking comes down to what's quickest and easiest, which is why it

can be so difficult to break away from the sort of food that isn't always what is best for you. I wanted to show that healthy food can be convenient as well as tasting good.

A key part of this is the ingredients you use. I generally stick with a few core things which I buy every week, which are versatile and fresh, and then add variety where I fancy. Generally I like to keep the list of items I buy regularly fairly short, supplemented by a few cupboard staples that require a one-off shop at a large supermarket or online order. Lots of fresh food is important too, and can be bought in most smaller shops and markets.

I know that, being based in London, I have a slightly biased perception of accessibility. I can source almost every ingredient I ever need from my local supermarket, and also have small independent healthfood shops just down the road that stock a few other ingredients I like to use. When I started out eating more

'I generally stick with a few core things which I buy every week, which are versatile and fresh, and then add variety when and where I fancy.'

healthily I didn't have the same local options for buying some of my staples, so I ordered a lot of things like tins of beans without stabilizers, tamari (gluten-free soy sauce) and bulk quantities of nuts online. Now, just a few years later, so much has changed in London that I can buy all of the above nearby. You will be familiar, I'm sure, with most of the ingredients mentioned in this book, but for a few that are a little more unusual I have included some short introductions. You can buy any of them online or in most healthfood shops, and most of them will last a long time so you don't have to budget for them regularly. I often buy things in bulk, which helps keep the cost down, too; I also do shop around for the best prices where possible as they can vary hugely.

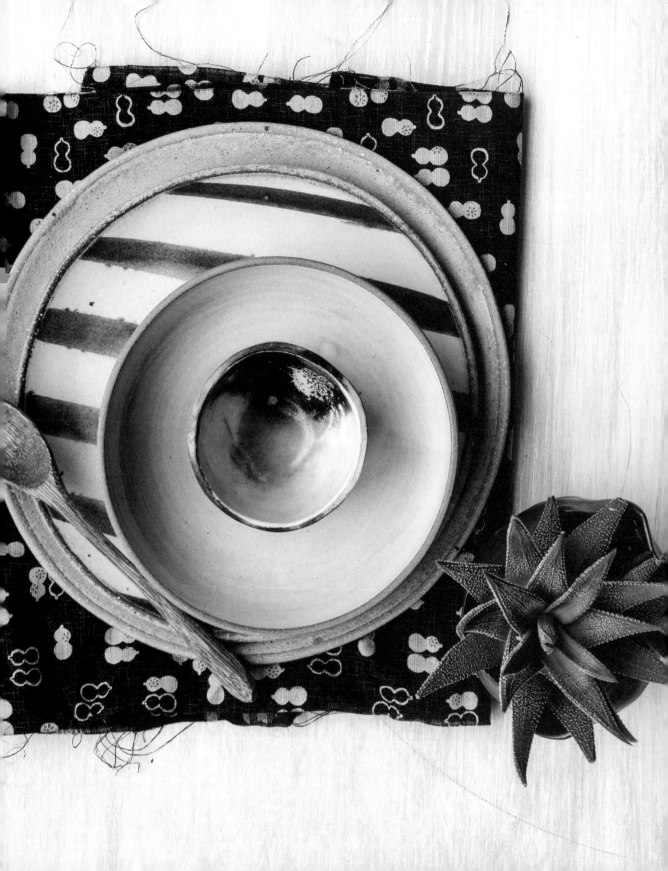

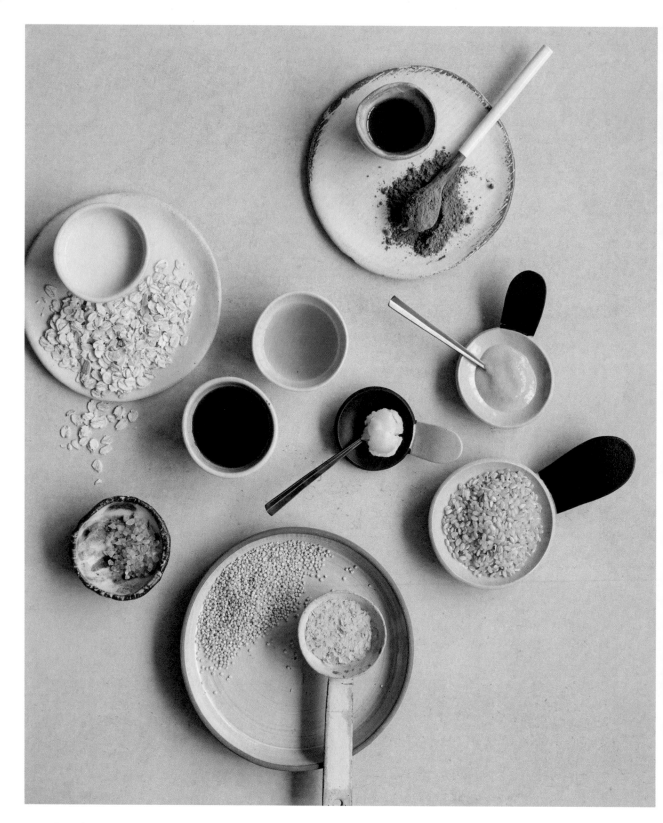

Cupboard Staples Explained

+ <u>Tamari</u>

This is a gluten-free soy sauce that I use in a lot of my cooking. I prefer it to salt and it's great for making sauces and dressings. If you are not excluding gluten from your diet, then regular soy sauce is fine, but watch out for hidden sugar in some brands. In most cases, salt or brown rice miso paste are also great alternatives.

+ <u>Tahini</u>

Tahini is a little like nut butter but made from sesame seeds. I choose light tahini where the sesame seeds have been hulled first to remove the skins, as it's less bitter than dark tahini. Again, this is great for sauces and dressings and it adds a creamy texture.

+ Apple Cider Vinegar

Apple cider vinegar (ACV) is a little sweeter than most other vinegars, as it is made from apples, as you may have guessed. It makes a great addition to dressings and salad dishes, and gives some added flavour to grains (just add a little to the cooking water as they boil).

There is a long list of proposed health benefits of ACV, including stabilizing blood sugar levels and helping to keep you full between meals. Always opt for natural or raw ACV, often labelled as 'with the mother' – you can identify it by its brown, murky colour and the stringy solids in the bottle. Some ACV has been filtered and processed, which removes some of the goodness, so while the processed kind still adds flavour to recipes, you may miss out on some of the health benefits.

+ Brown Rice Vinegar

Brown rice vinegar I use less often, but it's a good one to have in the cupboard and its shelf-life is so long that you can keep it for ages and use it bit by bit. Like ACV, it has a sweetness to it and the acidity is less aggressive than with other traditional vinegars.

+ Coconut Oil

Coconut oil is a real staple for me. It is so much more readily available than a few years ago. Always try to opt for raw, virgin coconut oil, which is the unprocessed form. It is more expensive but far superior in terms of health benefits than a cheaper alternative. Again, it will last forever in your cupboard so you won't have to keep shelling out for it every week. I try to buy a couple of jars when it's on offer to save a little on cost where possible, and it will usually last me a long time. It has many, many uses in a number of different recipes and cooking styles.

+ Sesame Oil

I use sesame oil for its flavour. I think it adds a great, nutty taste to dishes so I often use it over olive oil in my cooking. You can, of course, use these two oils interchangeably, but do note that your choice will affect the taste – which is why I will have selected one over the other in the recipes in this book.

+ Nutritional Yeast

Not only does this one sound strange but it looks pretty odd, too. Nutritional yeast is a deactivated yeast and looks a little like fish food! It usually comes in flakes and adds a really great cheesy flavour to dishes such as mac and 'cheese'. It is also great to sprinkle on top of pasta dishes or mashed potato, or for flavouring kale chips and popcorn. It is a good source of some B vitamins and also provides a relatively high amount of protein per serving, making it a great addition to a vegetarian or vegan diet.

+ Pink Himalayan Salt

I like to use pink Himalayan salt as it has the closest mineral composition to that found in the body. It is also not processed, unlike table salt, and adds a richer flavour.

+ Quinoa

Quinoa is one of the few plant-based complete proteins, meaning that it contains all of the nine essential amino acids. It has a slightly nutty taste but is subtle enough to take on the flavour of whatever you are cooking it with, so it works well in many different styles of dishes.

+ Short-grain Brown Rice

I generally buy short-grain brown rice – mainly for its texture. It isn't refined like white rice, and the extra fibre stops the blood sugar from spiking. Regular brown rice is great too and is more readily available than short-grain.

+ Oats

I use oats a lot – they are pretty versatile and are a great way of adding slow-release carbohydrates to meals. For a while I bought gluten-free oats, not realizing that oats themselves don't actually contain gluten. The difference between regular oats and gluten-free oats is the certification, meaning that gluten-free oats have no chance of contamination by gluten during the production process. For most people who struggle to digest gluten, regular oats are fine, but for coeliacs it is always recommended to buy the certified gluten-free variety. In my experience the majority of those with gluten intolerances are fine with regular oats. That said, there is something else in oats that can actually cause problems in some people: oats contain a protein that is similar to gluten, and there are some who have a specific problem digesting it. I think this is where some of the confusion comes from. Experiment, stick with it to let your body adjust, and see what works for you.

I like to buy jumbo oats – they add a much better texture to things like porridge, as you can soak them for a few minutes beforehand to make them go lovely and creamy.

+ Milk Alternatives

I tend to use brown rice milk, oat milk and almond milk at home – brown rice milk is sweeter so great for porridge and hot drinks. For savoury recipes, I like almond milk best.

When buying plant-based milk it is really important to check the ingredients, as there are lots on the market which contain unnatural additives and ingredients. There are some really great brands around and it is getting much easier to pick up dairy alternatives. Most of them can be stored in a cupboard until opening, so I tend to pick up a few at a time to keep me going, which is also great if you can't grab it locally.

+ Kitchen Equipment

People often ask what kind of kitchen equipment you need in order to be healthy. The real answer is none, and so please do not be put off when you see recipes calling for food processors, blenders or anything else. While there are a few things that you won't be able to make if you don't have the right equipment, most of the recipes in this book don't call for anything special.

Food processors are different from blenders. Blenders have a fine blade and require a little liquid in order to get things going. They are great for smoothies, sauces, soups and dressings. For hummus, nut butter, energy balls and more solid recipes, I like to use a food processor. You can now get blenders that are capable of doing both types of mixing, so it is worth doing your research to find out what suits you best. Equipment is bulky and good ones can be pricey. I started off with a 2-in-1 which had one base and then an interchangeable food processor/blender which was a really great, more affordable and space-saving solution while I was still getting to grips with my new way of cooking and eating. Over time I upgraded, but you should definitely shop around to find something that works best for you.

Spiralizers are great fun – I love having the option to quickly make spaghetti out of courgettes, carrots or whatever other vegetables I fancy. However, they wouldn't be the first thing I'd rush out and buy. They aren't expensive when you compare them to a blender or food processor, but they can be bulky and awkward to store. You can get handheld ones but their use is limited. Alternatively you can use a peeler to make ribbons instead of noodles – which works really well, too!

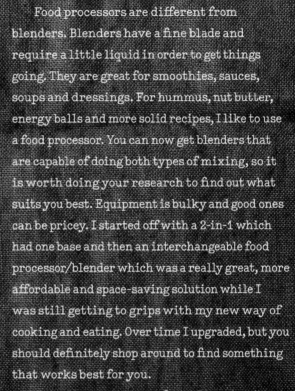

A Little on Nutrition

Superfoods

By definition, a superfood is 'A nutrient-rich food considered to be especially beneficial for health and well-being' (*Oxford English Dictionary*), and they are really having their moment. 'Superfood' has become a bit of a marketing buzzword but these foods do serve a useful purpose in supplementing a healthy diet. Importantly, they should complement a varied, healthy diet of nutritious foods, rather than be relied on as a substitute for fresh, whole foods.

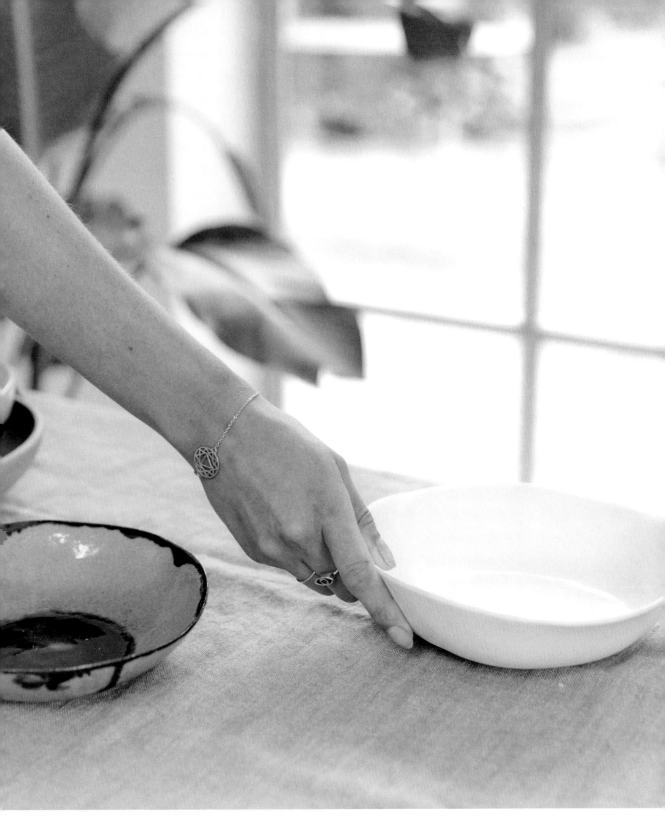

Bowl

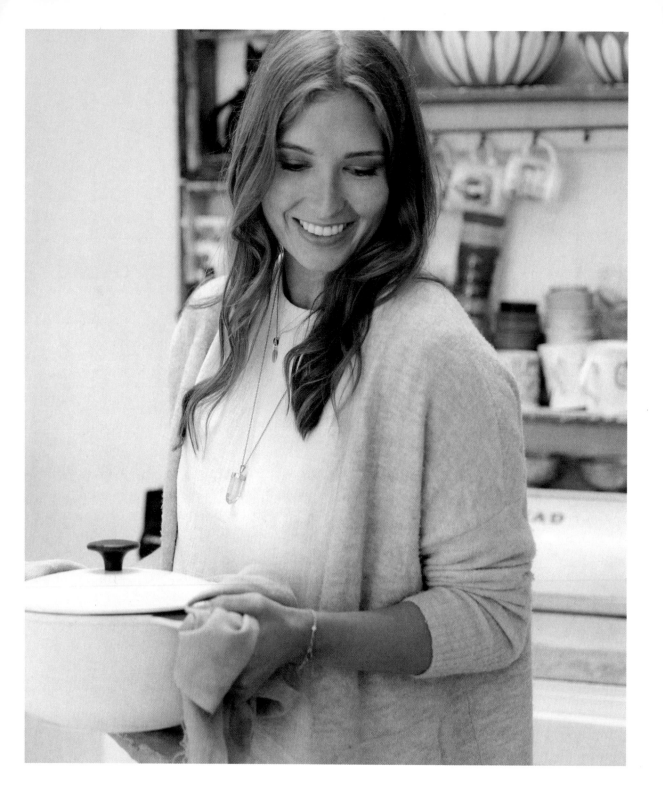

For those who have the disposable income available to spend on an array of powders, then by all means include these in your daily diet if you choose. But you really don't need to splash out to eat healthily. You may actually already be eating superfoods without realizing it – everyday foods which are truly 'super' include kale, blueberries and oats.

If you do want an added boost, don't feel compelled to buy everything you hear about. In my experience you'll end up with a cupboard full of expired powders. Pick one or two, opting for smaller packets to begin with, and stick with those. See if they improve how you feel and are easy enough to use. If they work for you then keep them up, if not, move on without worrying about it.

Calories

Essentially, the important thing to remember is that if we take in more calories than we burn, it can cause us to gain weight as we store the excess in our bodies. In the same way, if we burn more than we consume, the opposite can happen. The trouble with calories is that they don't correspond to the nutritional value of a food type. So something that is low-calorie isn't necessarily healthy, and may well contain a lot of other ingredients that you may wish to avoid.

Calorie-counting is a popular tool for controlling weight, and for many it is incredibly effective. It can be a useful way to be mindful of the quantities you are eating but it can also become an obsession and dangerous for certain people. As a teenager I spent time obsessing over the maths, making sure I didn't exceed a certain limit that I had set myself each day.

What I think is really important to understand is that not all calories are equal. You could compare an avocado and a chocolate bar, or a banana and a packet of sweets, a homemade hearty meal and something pre-made from the supermarket – the calorie content might be the same, but the list of ingredients – and the health benefits – will be very different.

What our bodies require varies hugely from day to day and week to week. Setting a target calorie intake means that you are not necessarily listening to your body. Some days you might be hungrier than others, or need a little more energy. Maybe you had a busier day or worked out more. Rather than punishing yourself and trying to stick to a certain number, I would urge you to base the quantities you eat on the way that you feel, and to drop the notion of calories where possible. When you begin to eat well, calories naturally seem less important anyway. You can over- or under-eat no matter what you are eating, but by bringing your focus to nutritious, fresh, healthy food and moving away from processed food, it becomes easier to find a balanced natural weight.

For me, once I was eating the right sorts of food, I totally ditched any sort of calorie-counting and was able to stop measuring what I was eating on a day-to-day basis. Thinking of it as a lifestyle rather than a diet made it a lot more sustainable and less all-consuming. I love the philosophy of thinking about filling yourself with as much natural goodness as possible and getting a good array of colours onto your plate. I now focus on variety, flavour and enjoying good food, rather than worrying about being too measured about it.

There is a fine line, of course: it is easy to be greedy and to eat more than you need, especially if you love food. I am certainly one of those people and often find myself eating without being hungry. My mealtimes mostly come around through routine rather than hunger. Being mindful about when and how much you eat can help you to listen more to your body. Slowing down also helps to prevent overeating. All of these things are helpful, but the real message here is to focus on finding good foods that offer a well-rounded and balanced diet.

Sugar

Sugar can be hidden in almost any type of food – even regular items like bread can be packed with it. Our bodies store excess sugar as fat, and many people are consuming a lot more sugar than they realize, which can contribute to weight gain as well as a whole host of other health problems.

It is found in processed foods, bread, confectionery, ready meals, and even salad dressings, and is incredibly addictive. The large amount of sugar regularly found in processed food is particularly bad for our bodies because it creates huge blood sugar spikes, which then come crashing back down, causing our energy levels to drop. The alternative is unrefined sugars, which are in their natural form. They take longer to reach the blood and the energy they contain is released more gradually.

I have learned that refined sugar doesn't suit me, leading to severe energy dips and stomach aches. Although unrefined sugars such as honey, date syrup, coconut sugar or maple syrup still affect our blood sugar levels, they can offer other nutritional benefits, so I opt for these over a refined alternative when I do use a sweetener.

The sugars in fruit are combined with the natural fibre in the fruit and therefore they have less of an effect on blood sugar levels. Fruit also contains a lot of other nutrients that keep us healthy, so while some people choose to cut out fruit when they go 'sugar-free', for me fruit makes up an important part of a balanced diet. That being said, I went through a period where bananas were sending my gut bacteria off-balance, so I took them out of my fruit bowl for a while. Just remember, it's about working out what makes your body feel good and adapting what you eat to suit it best.

Fat

Lots of people seem to be scared of including fats in their diets. There is a huge difference in how various types of fats impact our bodies. The term 'low fat' can also be quite misleading. A lot of 'fat-free' food can be higher in other things to add flavour, such as sugar, additives or refined carbohydrates, which leaves us questioning whether they are actually healthier or not.

There are many debates around this topic, but the take-home message is that you need some fats to help your body absorb certain vitamins. These fats are called 'essential' because the body is unable to produce them; they can be found in foods such as avocados, olives, nuts and seeds. They are also really wonderful for your hair and skin, helping to give you that healthy glow.

Protein

Your body needs protein for growth and repair, so it is essential that you get enough in your diet. There are lots of different sources of protein – meat, fish and eggs being the obvious choices, but there are also plenty of plant-based protein sources. Those following a vegetarian or vegan diet, or even those who just want to reduce their intake of animal produce, don't have to suffer by not getting enough protein in their diets.

Proteins are formed of different amino acid chains, some of which your body is able to produce. The ones that your body cannot make itself are called essential amino acids, and these are the ones you need in your diet.

There are nine essential amino acids. A complete protein source contains all of these essential amino acids. The most obvious source is animal protein. While you can get protein from non-animal sources, these are often incomplete proteins, which means that variety is incredibly important in order

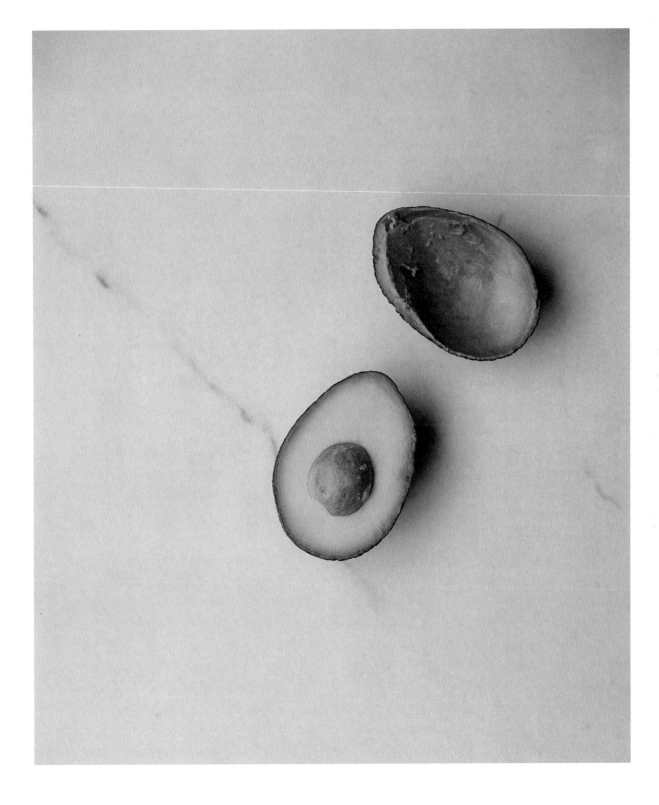

Bowl

to make sure you get a full range over the course of a few days or a week.

I think we can all agree that, as with anything you put into your body, the less processed, the better. I tend to avoid processed meat substitutes, as they often contain funny ingredients or additives that I like to steer clear of. This comes down to personal preference again, but now that I have spent time learning about my body, I no longer feel the need to substitute in that way. As with all packaged food, checking the ingredients list is a good habit to get into, as it helps you choose the foods that work best for you.

I choose not to eat meat, because that's what makes me feel best, and I have also become more conscious of how my lifestyle impacts on the environment. Some people feel best when they include meat in their diet, and of course I believe you should do what works for you. I would, however, encourage meat-eaters to buy better-quality meat (organic and free-range), even if this means reducing the frequency of meat-based meals to make it work within your budget.

Carbohydrates

Lots of people also have a negative association with carbs, thanks to the popularity of certain well-known diet plans. Cutting carbs seems to be a go-to diet for many, but really what does it do to your body?

Especially for those of you who like to be active, carbohydrates are essential as they are your main energy source. The body has a limited ability to store carbs, so eating small portions regularly keeps the levels topped up; this means that you have the energy you need to go about your daily life and take part in exercise and physical activity. While you do get energy from fats and proteins, cutting carbohydrates can cause imbalances and energy deficiency.

Carbohydrates are made up of sugars, starches and fibre. Focus where possible on wholegrain, starchy carbs rather than high-sugar foods and, where necessary, pay attention to portion size rather than completely eliminating this food group from your diet.

Gluten

Gluten is a protein that can be difficult for some people to digest. It is found in many different grains such as wheat, rye and barley. While there is much debate on the subject, it has been suggested that the modification of crops has led to an increase in sensitivity to gluten. While some people have no trouble with gluten, many others have symptoms such as digestive issues, skin irritation, fatigue and aching joints, which may be relieved by reducing their gluten intake.

It can take a little while to notice a difference when experimenting with gluten. If you are planning on giving it up for a bit, I would recommend trying for several weeks before assessing the impact that it has on you. You do not need to buy expensive free-from products (these tend to be high in sugar and packed with unwelcome ingredients anyway), simply choose other grains such as brown rice and quinoa, which are naturally gluten-free.

Once you are more in touch with your own body, there are options such as rye and spelt, which contain lower levels of gluten than wheat flour, which you can experiment with. I found it really interesting to introduce these back into my diet and to keep an eye on what worked for me. Nowadays I find that I can have rye every now and then, but if I eat it too often then my symptoms start to return. It's handy to know this in case I get stuck out and about without anything to eat, as it's fairly readily available. Again, it's about understanding your body and making life as easy for yourself as possible.

Dairy

I've spent a lot of time reading about the impact of different foods on the body. Personally I have always had trouble digesting dairy; as a child it left me with eczema and I grew up drinking goat's milk. As an adult, even goat's milk dairy products began to give me digestive issues, and so eventually I decided it had to go, too.

I was pretty devastated at the idea – I've never been a big milk drinker, but cheese was a firm favourite for me.

Many people may notice a difference in their digestion, skin and mood by cutting out dairy, and there are many studies suggesting that we should all try it. Like anything, this comes down to each of our bodies and finding what works for us individually. Even if dairy doesn't seem to impact you negatively, you may want to reduce your consumption due to concerns over animal welfare or the environmental impact of dairy farming. The great thing is that plant-based alternatives are becoming more easily available; I would just encourage you to read the labels to avoid anything over-processed. Almond milk or oat milk are really easy to make yourself, too, so if you really want to make sure you are sticking to the good stuff, that's a really great option. It definitely helped me when I first started and couldn't find good branded products very easily.

Additives and Preservatives

While ideally we would all eat 100 per cent fresh food all the time, it may not be realistic or practical and we need things that come in packets and tins, such as kidney beans and chickpeas, to get a well-rounded nutritional intake. If you are looking to reduce your intake of additives and preservatives, getting into the habit of checking the ingredients lists on labels can be really helpful. For example, when buying dried fruit, I always look for the packets that haven't got lots of preservatives – the apricots may look browner but they won't be preserved with unnecessary chemicals.

Alcohol

Whether or not we choose to drink alcohol can depend on lots of different factors and, like everything, this should be a personal decision. If drinking is a central part of how you socialize with friends, it can be hard to

'You are allowed, or in fact strongly encouraged, to do what makes you happy. That is what this is all about – making it work for you.'

consider ditching that altogether – and besides, it may not be something that you ever want to do. Once you start looking at other areas of your life, it may be that you decide you would rather not drink as much or as frequently, if you find that it prevents you from feeling good. Perhaps drinking alcohol will become something you save for special occasions, or maybe you will change the type of alcohol that you drink. Or it might be that you don't want to change anything here at all. As always, you need to find what works best for you.

Try not to allow other people's judgement to get in the way of what you decide with regards to drinking, or in fact any other part of your lifestyle. People will always have something to say, but don't let that affect your choices.

Remember, it is about finding your balance. If you enjoy going out and having a drink then I, for one, am not telling you not to. You are allowed, or in fact strongly encouraged, to do what makes you happy. That is what this is all about – making it work for you.

'Bowl' Round-up

The food that you eat has a big effect on how you feel. By choosing to fill yourself with healthy fuel that you respond well to, you can help your body to be its most efficient, enabling you to feel energetic, light and clear-minded. Of course, it is just one pillar in the 'trio of wellness', but in some cases it is the most essential one in terms of feeling our best. We could all follow the same diet and each of us could end up feeling completely different. By tuning in to your body and starting to recognize how different foods and eating habits make you feel, you can familiarize yourself with what works for you and adapt your meals accordingly. It is important to use your body to guide you in the right direction for you. Be mindful about how you eat and become conscious of any bad habits you may have developed over time. Acknowledge patterns such as emotional eating if they exist for you, and find ways to address and overcome them as you learn more and more about yourself.

When we tie together Mind, Body and Bowl in a way that works for us as individuals, we can create a lifestyle that suits what we need physically, mentally and emotionally.

By taking inspiration from those around you and then, crucially, adapting it to suit yourself, taking and leaving the bits that do and do not work, you can create your own version of balance. But it all starts with learning about yourself, shifting away from anything negative and letting go of whatever may be holding you back from your true self. Establish your values, work out how to bring them into each part of your life and grow in the direction that you wish to see yourself. Find support in the networks that really understand who you are, release the need to conform to your own and other people's expectations. Learn to embrace positivity as a way of life, and find comfort in the transience of everything around you. Do what makes your soul happy and have fun trying to figure out what that may be. Change is natural and exciting, so learn to embrace it. Finally, allow yourself to make mistakes. Enjoy every imperfection, knowing that they make you the perfect version of yourself.

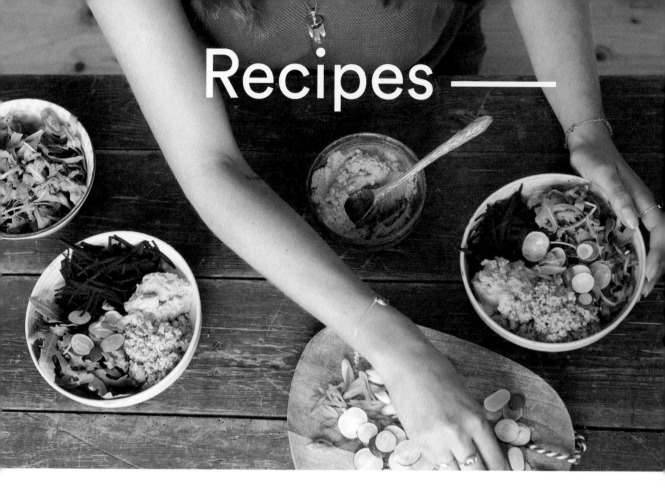

Recipes

In this section you will find nearly 60 recipes designed to help you include simple, healthy and delicious food in your lifestyle. All the recipes are dairy, gluten and refined-sugar free and are also entirely plant-based in order to make them suitable to as many people as possible. I like to eat this way all the time. It is what makes me feel best and these are the ingredients, flavours and dishes that I love. But these can just serve as ideas for you to build upon, add to and to inspire you to cook simple, fresh food at home. I hope you find some things you love and that you can share them with your friends and family. Remember, it all comes down to simplicity, convenience and what works for you. Most importantly, I hope you enjoy them as part of your own balanced, healthy and happy lifestyle, created by you, for you, and that this helps you to feel the best version of yourself.

01

simple
healthy
delicious
breakfasts
best start
to the day

Blueberry Overnight Oats

Overnight oats are such a great breakfast for anyone who finds themselves in a rush to leave the house in the morning or for those of us who are up and out before we are ready for breakfast. Everything is prepared the night before in just a few minutes, sealed and popped in the fridge, ready to grab on your way out the door.

Overnight oats are also a great alternative when you don't feel like hot porridge, and a smoothie won't hit the spot. This recipe includes hemp seeds to boost the protein content, but if you don't have any at home it is still a nutritious breakfast without them.

60g blueberries
50g jumbo oats
20g shelled hemp
seeds – optional
¼ tsp vanilla powder
(or ½ tsp honey)
150ml almond milk

Place the blueberries in a small pan with 50ml boiling water over a low heat. As they begin to warm, use the back of a spoon to gently squash the blueberries. Once the water has been bubbling for a minute or so and has turned a deep purple, remove from the heat and pour the blueberries into a small bowl to cool.

In a glass jar, combine the oats, hemp seeds (if using), vanilla powder or honey and mix together. Then add the almond milk and 50ml cold water. Use a spoon to make sure the liquid gets to the bottom of the jar.

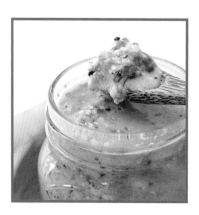

Once the blueberries have cooled, pour them into the jar with any remaining juices. Stir through the oats and then seal with a lid. Give the jar a good shake, then place in the fridge ready to soak overnight (or for an hour or two).

Cinnamon, Apple and Raisin Porridge

When I first started eating porridge, I loved topping it with raisins and an apple compote. I still make porridge almost every day but don't often have the foresight to prepare the apple in advance for mornings when I'm short of time.

This recipe is a bit of a shortcut, which achieves all the amazing flavours that I love so much but without having to plan ahead.

Place the apple chunks in a saucepan with 200ml boiling water and the cinnamon. Heat over a medium heat for 5 minutes or until the apples start to soften.

Turn off the heat and add the oats and raisins or sultanas. Stir well to make sure they are totally covered by the liquid and leave to soak for 5–10 minutes until the oats are soft and plump and have absorbed most of the liquid.

Pour the milk into the pan and cook the porridge over a medium-low heat.

Stir often for 8 minutes or until the oats have absorbed the liquid and you have your desired consistency.

1 apple, peeled, cored and cut into chunks
1 tsp ground cinnamon
45g jumbo oats
20g raisins or sultanas
100ml brown rice milk or nut milk

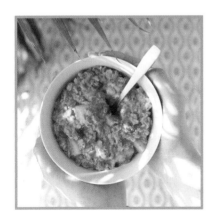

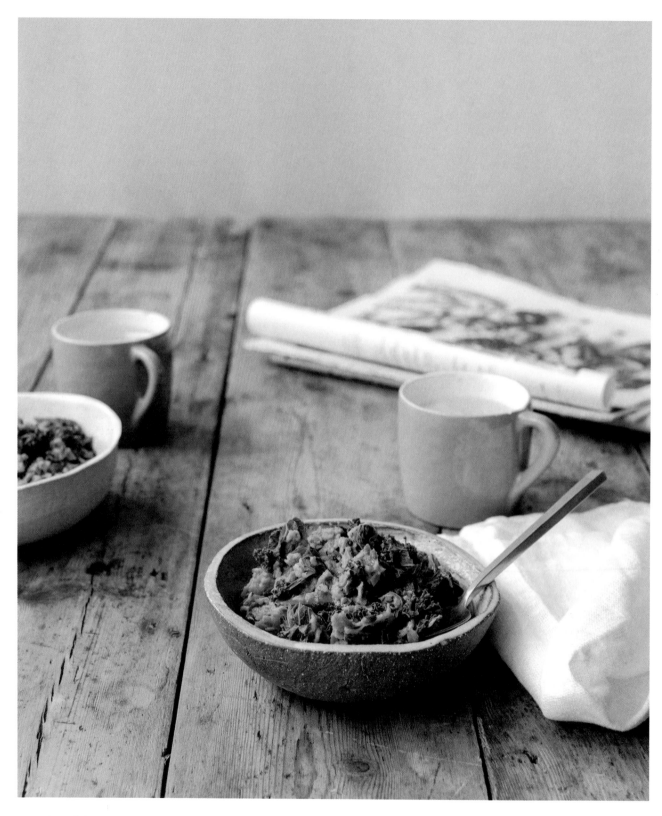

Savoury Porridge

This risotto or savoury porridge may sound a little strange, but I only had to experiment with it once to be totally converted! It doesn't have to be confined to breakfast – I often make it in the evenings if I want something quick and warming.

Begin by making the stock. Place the miso and mixed herbs in 1 litre boiling water and whisk well until the paste has totally dissolved, then set to one side.

In a large saucepan, heat the olive oil over a medium–low heat and add the garlic. Stir well to make sure it does not burn. Then add the onion and allow it to soften slightly before mixing in the leek. Leave to sweat for 5 minutes. I like to season generously with pepper here, but the stock is already salty so I would wait until the end to add any extra.

Once the leek and onion are soft, add the mushrooms. Stir in for 1 minute and then add the kale, using your hands to break it into small pieces if needed.

Once the mushrooms are turning brown and the kale has softened, after about 7 minutes, stir in the oats to coat them in any juices and oil in the pan.

Give the stock another stir to reincorporate anything that has sunk to the bottom. Then start to add the stock to the oats, a third at a time, and stir well. Leave to simmer for 15–20 minutes until the liquid has absorbed, stirring occasionally to break up any lumps. Once the stock has been absorbed and the oats are soft, the porridge is ready.

1 tbsp olive oil
2 garlic cloves, crushed
1 onion, diced
1 large leek, quartered
    lengthways and
    finely sliced
200g mushrooms,
    stalks removed
    and finely sliced
100g kale, thick
    stalks removed
200g jumbo oats
salt and pepper

For the stock
2 tbsp brown rice
    miso paste
2 tsp dried
    mixed herbs

Black Rice Porridge with Pear Compote

I love this recipe because it is different from anything I've ever really tried before. I don't know where the idea came from – possibly I saw a black rice and pear salad on a menu somewhere and it then evolved in my mind. But it's a winner, especially if you feel like something a little fancier at breakfast but without having to put the work in.

Not only does it look good, but it's also full of flavour. The rice has a lovely consistency and the pears, done in two different ways, add to that by offering a bit of sweetness, too.

For the porridge
140g Thai black rice
100ml almond milk
a pinch of salt

For the compote
2½ pears, peeled, cored and roughly chopped
1 tsp coconut sugar
3 cardamom pods

For the topping
½ pear
2 tsp coconut sugar
½ tsp ground cardamom

Start by boiling the rice in 400ml water, cover with a lid and reduce to a simmer. It takes 35–40 minutes to cook, so you can leave it going while you make the compote, just checking on it occasionally. Remove the lid after 20 minutes so that the water starts to simmer off.

Place the pears for the compote in a second pan with 150ml boiling water and the coconut sugar. Crush the cardamom pods with the back of a knife and scoop out the seeds, adding them to the pan. Once the pears have softened, after 10 minutes, drain the water into the pan of rice and then mash or blend the pears into a smooth compote.

Preheat the oven to 180°C/350°F/Gas Mark 4.

Cut the pear for the topping into long slices, 5mm thick. In a small bowl, mix 25ml boiling water with the coconut sugar and ground cardamom. Line a baking tray with baking parchment and arrange the slices of pear on top. Then drizzle over the coconut and cardamom syrup and bake for 5 minutes or until the pears brown slightly. Remove from the oven and place to one side.

Once the rice has almost cooked, add the almond milk and salt, then stir through until you have a loose, porridge-like consistency. The rice should still have some texture to it but it should look creamy rather than watery.

Divide the porridge between two bowls, topping with the compote and the baked pears to serve.

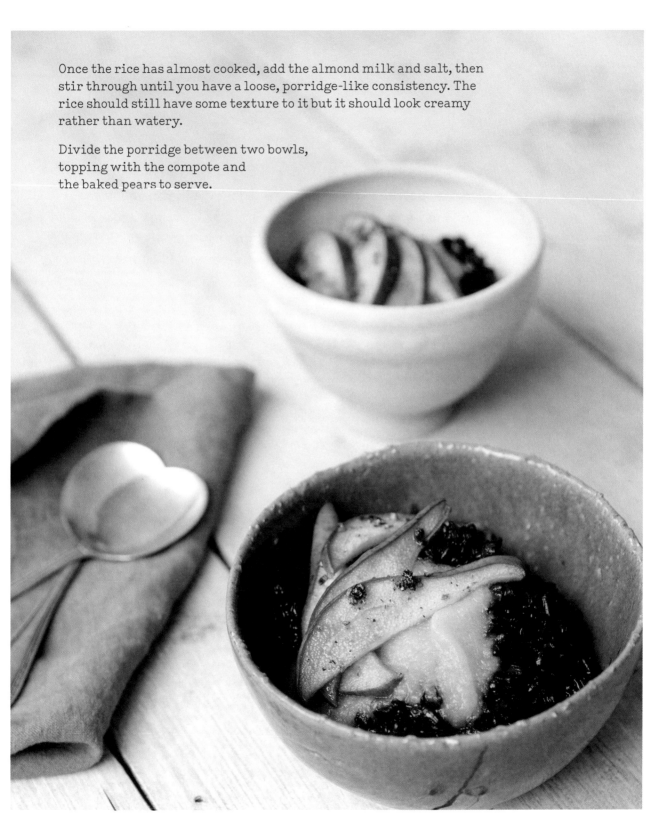

Chocolate Chip Granola

This granola is so delicious with a banana-based smoothie bowl, coconut yoghurt or just on its own as a snack. It will even turn your almond milk chocolaty and offers a more nutritious take on a shop-bought chocolate breakfast cereal.

125g almonds
200g jumbo oats
70ml coconut oil
10g raw cacao
  powder
45ml date syrup
35ml maple syrup
60g cacao nibs

Preheat the oven to 150°C/300°F/Gas Mark 2.

Start by breaking up the almonds either in a food processor or by roughly chopping, then add them to a mixing bowl with the oats.

Heat the coconut oil gently in a pan, then pour over the oats and almonds. Add the cacao powder, date syrup and maple syrup, and stir well until everything is evenly coated. Then add the cacao nibs and mix thoroughly.

Spread the granola in a thin layer on a large baking tray and place in the oven for 45 minutes or until crispy, stirring regularly to prevent it from burning, especially at the corners.

Remove the granola from the trays and allow to cool completely before transferring it to an airtight container, where it can be stored for up to 2 weeks.

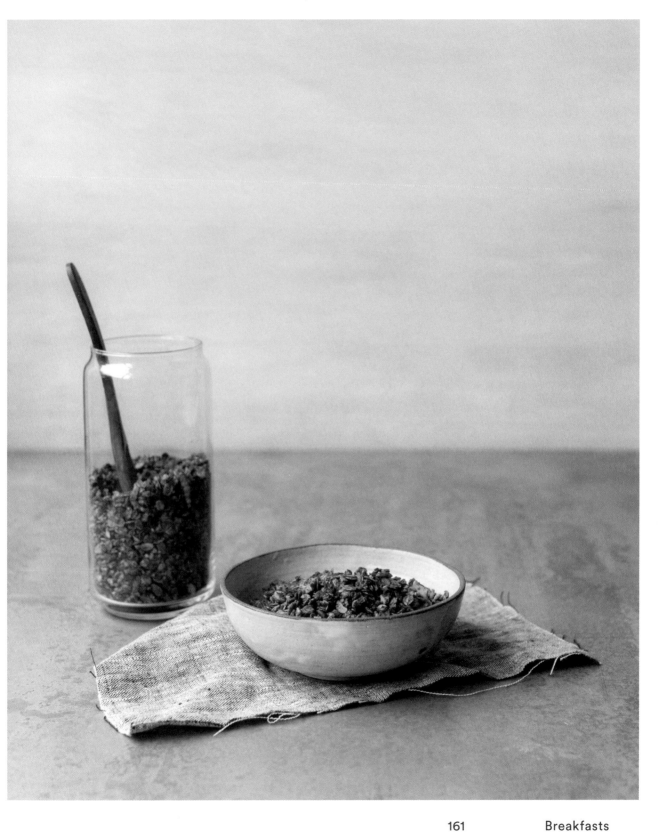

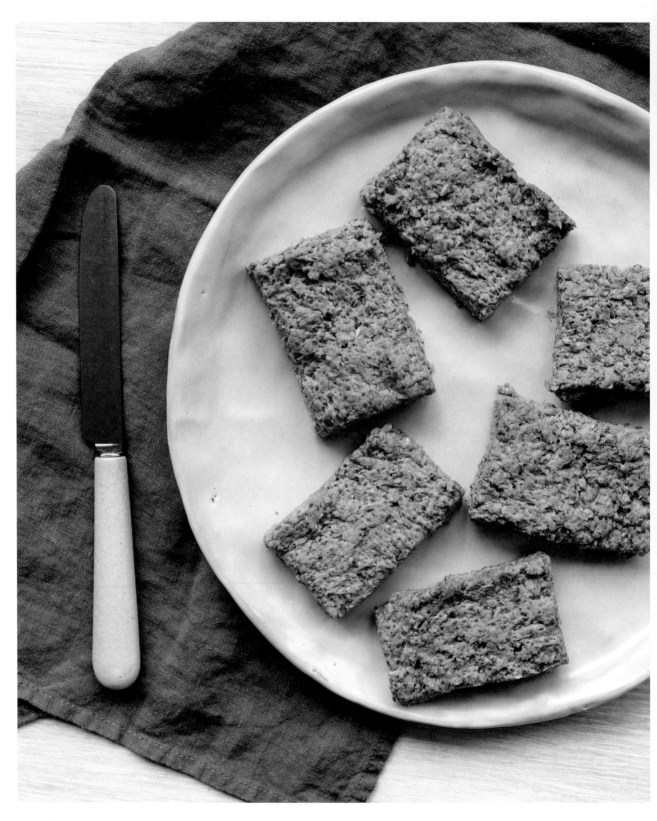

Banana and Raspberry No-Bake Breakfast Bars

Makes 6 bars

These bars are perfect for when you are on the go. Plus they set in the freezer so you don't have to bake them, meaning they only take 5 minutes to make!

Not overly sweet, their flavour comes from the banana and raspberry. They are great to grab on the way out the door on a busy morning or if you are looking for something to keep you going during the day.

Combine the raspberries and 50ml water in a small saucepan over a medium–low heat and cover with the lid for a few minutes, until they start to break down. Add the chia seeds, starting with 3 tablespoons, and stir well. Leave the mixture to one side to form a gel, adding extra chia seeds if needed to absorb excess liquid.

In a food processor, mix the oats, peanut butter and banana, then transfer the mixture to a bowl. Stir in the raspberry chia gel.

Line a small baking tray (16 x 26cm) with baking parchment, leaving some hanging over the sides to make it easier to lift the bars out later. Tip in the mixture and use a spatula to spread it evenly. Then place it in the freezer for at least 1 hour. Once set, use a sharp knife to cut the mixture into bars (or squares if you want something more snack-size).

The bars can then be stored, covered, in the freezer for 1 week, or for a few days in the fridge.

100g frozen raspberries
3–4 tbsp chia seeds
100g jumbo oats
100g peanut butter
1 banana

Raspberry Tahini Porridge

This is such a creamy porridge bowl, combining two of my favourite flavours to give an indulgent but healthy breakfast that will keep you going on a busy day. The tahini contains healthy fats, while the oats provide you with slow-release carbohydrates for long-lasting energy.

50g jumbo oats
75g frozen raspberries
½ tsp coconut sugar
    (or maple syrup)
125ml almond milk
a small pinch of salt
1–2 tsp tahini, to taste
a pinch of sesame seeds

Soak the oats in a small pan with 200ml boiling water for 5 minutes.

In a second small pan, heat the raspberries with 25ml water over a medium-high heat, covering with a lid until the raspberries soften. Use the back of a spoon to squash the raspberries, then add the coconut sugar or maple syrup and stir occasionally, allowing the water to boil off gently. When the raspberries are totally broken down but not watery, turn off the hob and set the pan to one side.

After 5 minutes, once the oats have absorbed the water, pour in the almond milk and place over a low heat. Add the salt and stir regularly for 10 minutes or until the oats thicken into a fluffy porridge.

Top with the raspberries, drizzling over the tahini and sprinkling with sesame seeds to serve.

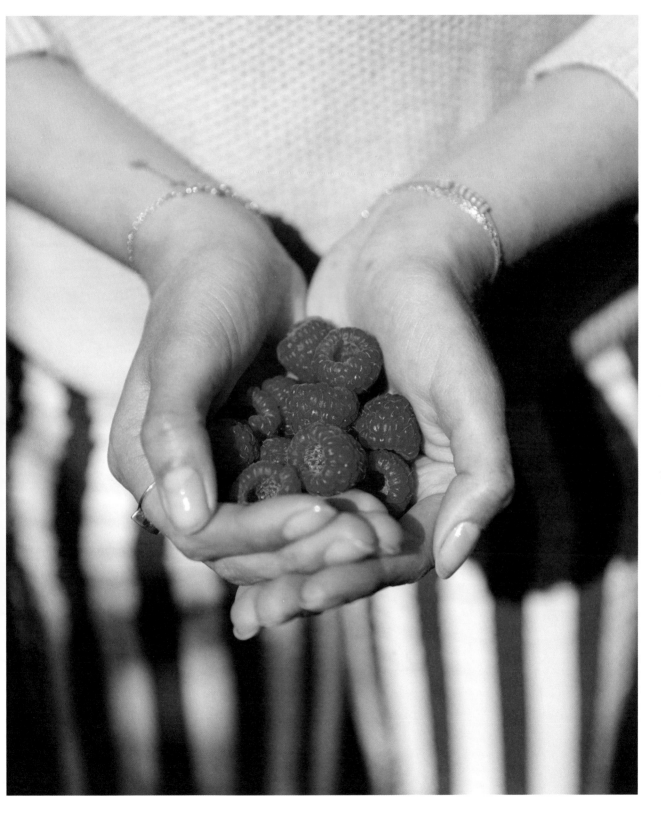

Breakfasts

Farmhouse Loaf

Delicious freshly baked bread is something that I've really missed since changing the way I eat. This loaf has helped me to fill that hole, and it works so well for sandwiches, toast or any other way you enjoy your bread.

100g chia seeds
200g oats or oat flour
115g buckwheat flour
3 tbsp sesame oil
2 tbsp honey
a pinch of salt
100ml almond milk

Preheat the oven to 160°C/315°F/Gas Mark 2½.

Place the chia seeds in a bowl with 200ml water, stir well and leave to soak for 5–10 minutes until a gel forms.

Place the oats in a food processor and blend until it forms a flour (you can skip this step if you are using oat flour).

Combine the oats, buckwheat flour and chia seed paste in a bowl and mix well. Then add the oil, honey and salt and fold them in. Slowly add the almond milk, bit by bit, until you have a dough that is sticky enough to hold together but doesn't stick to your hands. You can use a little more or less milk as necessary.

Line a baking tray with baking parchment, then use your hands to shape the dough into a loaf on top of the paper.

Place in the oven for 25 minutes, then turn it over and bake for a further 25 minutes. Finally, turn it once more and bake for 10 minutes or until the loaf starts to brown. Remove from the oven and allow to cool and set for a few minutes.

Store in an airtight container if you want the loaf to last more than a few days, or slice and then freeze.

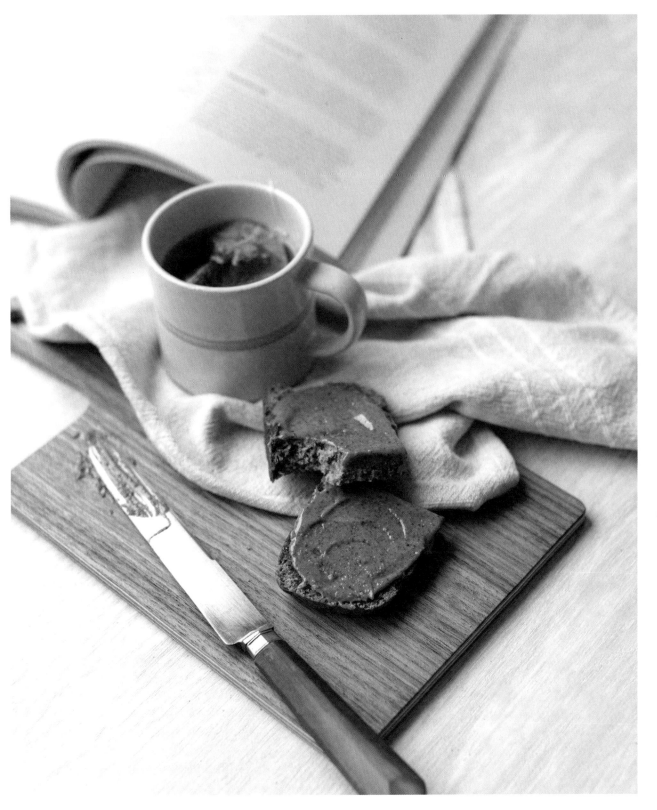

Cinnamon Buckwheat Granola

This recipe is really close to my heart. Back when I wasn't really sure what Mind Body Bowl was, I experimented with a few things, one of which was a brief stint producing granola. It happened completely by accident – I just decided to give it a go, throwing ingredients together one day at home, and it turned out better than I ever expected.

For the next few months, I made and sold batches to friends, friends of friends and so on, until I couldn't keep up with the orders. At which point, I had to make a decision: continue on a small scale, find investment and make a real shot of it or move on with the happy memory of making delicious granola.

I never shared the recipe, in case I decided to start up again, but my first book seems a good place to do so. I hope you enjoy it as much as I know so many others have, and thank you to those who tried it and helped me explore that idea when I was figuring things out. This is especially for you.

130g jumbo oats
175g untoasted
   buckwheat groats
30ml coconut oil
60ml maple syrup
1 tsp date syrup
   – optional
2 tsp ground cinnamon
170g almonds
100g raisins

Preheat the oven to 160°C/315°F/Gas Mark 2½.

In a mixing bowl, combine the oats and buckwheat.

Over a low heat, melt the coconut oil and mix in the maple and date (if using) syrups. Then remove from the heat and add the cinnamon, before pouring into the mixing bowl.

Line two large baking trays with baking parchment and spread the granola in an even layer. Place the granola in the oven and stir thoroughly every 10 minutes to make sure none of it burns.

Place the almonds in a food processor to break them into smaller chunks, being careful not to break them down too much.

Once the granola is golden brown (30–40 minutes), add the almonds and raisins, and bake for a further 5 minutes.

Remove the granola from the trays and allow to cool completely before transferring it to an airtight container, where it can be stored for up to a month.

Coconut and Mango Overnight Oats

This is such a fresh version of this easy breakfast, bringing a little sunshine to any morning. I love the combination of coconut and mango, it just reminds me of summer or takes me to a wonderful beach somewhere. If coconut is not your thing, then you can just leave it out and stick with mango.

1 ripe mango
200ml almond milk
80g jumbo oats
1 small packet (24g)
  coconut flakes

Cut the mango from either side of the large stone. Make cuts through the flesh in a crisscross pattern to the skin. Push the skin side inwards and use a knife to cut off the pieces of flesh. Then cut around the stone and peel the skin from the flesh. Place the mango flesh in a blender with the milk. Blend until smooth (although if you want to leave a few small chunks of mango for texture, that's a great way to do it, too!).

Pour the mango mix into a mixing bowl and stir in the oats.

Decant the mango oats evenly into two jars. Sprinkle half the coconut flakes on top of each and then seal. Place in the fridge overnight, ready for breakfast the next day. If the oats and liquid separate too much, just give the jar a shake to keep the consistency even and help the oats to absorb all the juicy mango.

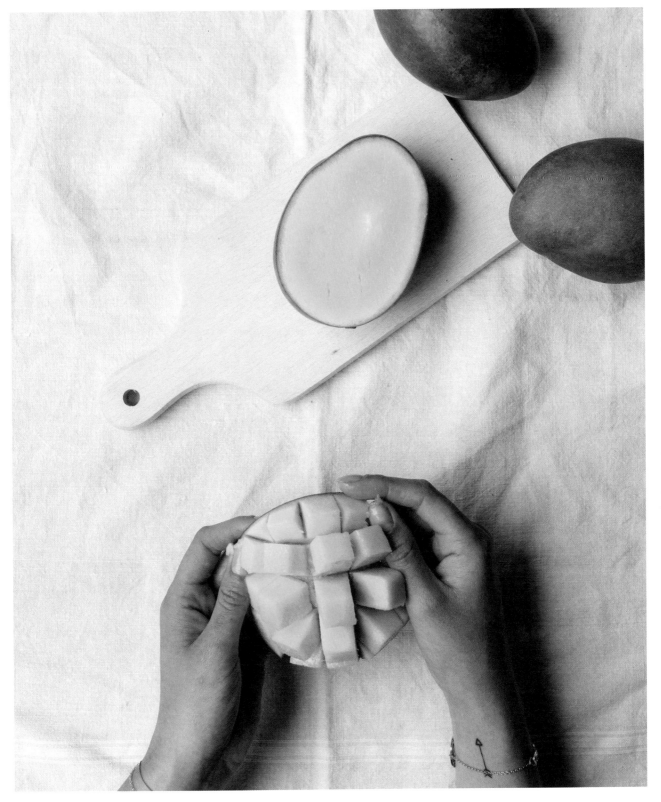

Breakfasts

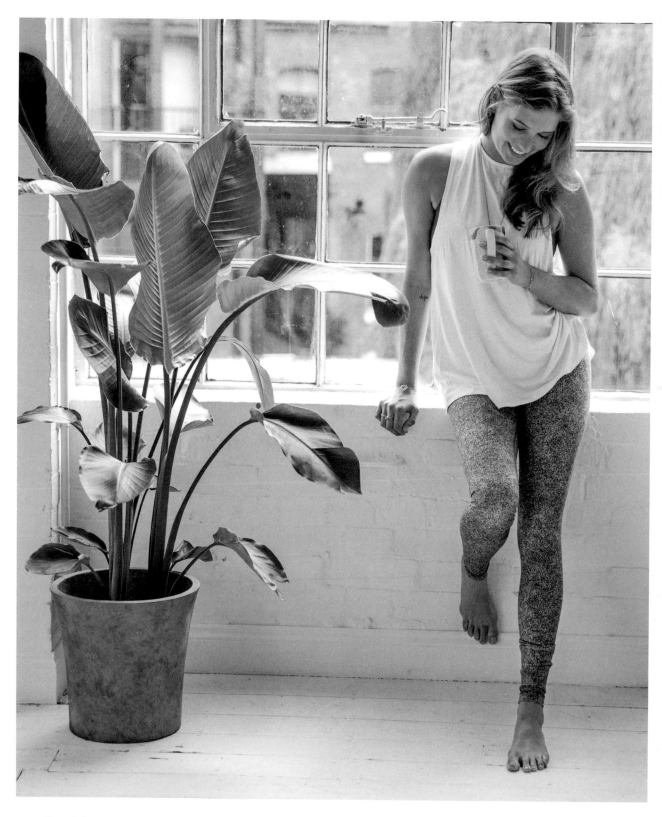

Spiced Quinoa Porridge

This recipe was inspired by a West Indian porridge that I became totally obsessed with on holiday a few summers ago. Every morning we were served a bowl of deliciously creamy and totally indulgent porridge cooked in coconut milk and spiced with bay leaves, star anise and sweetened with banana and honey. I can still remember the taste when I think back to it.

This is a lighter version I developed back home, still with a lot of flavour but a little less indulgent. The quinoa adds a little protein to the bowl and I make it with brown rice milk rather than coconut milk so that it isn't as rich. That said, if you do fancy something more authentic, you can always go for oats instead and use coconut milk, of course.

Place the quinoa in a pan with 150ml boiling water and begin to heat gently, stirring occasionally.

Once most of the water has been absorbed, which takes 7 minutes, add the bay leaf, 100ml of the brown rice milk, the nutmeg, the cinnamon and coconut oil, and stir well. Using the back of a knife, crush the cardamom pods and throw those in too.

Mix in the banana, adding the remaining 50ml rice milk and 50ml boiling water, and stir again. The quinoa should be totally soft and you can add extra milk or water if needed. Once you have a thickened but still runny consistency, remove the quinoa from the heat and take out the bay leaf and cardamom pods, then stir in the desiccated coconut.

Top with the roughly chopped almonds and sliced banana (or any other toppings of choice) to serve.

60g quinoa
1 bay leaf
150ml brown rice milk
¼ tsp freshly
    grated nutmeg
¼ tsp ground cinnamon
1 tsp coconut oil
2 cardamom pods
½ banana, chopped
10g desiccated coconut

Suggested toppings
15g almonds,
    roughly chopped
½ banana, sliced

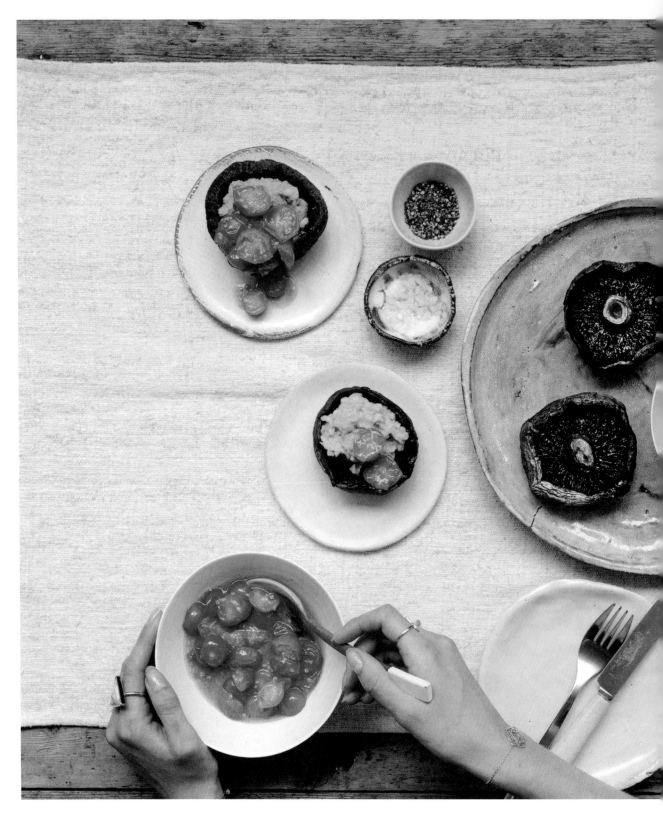

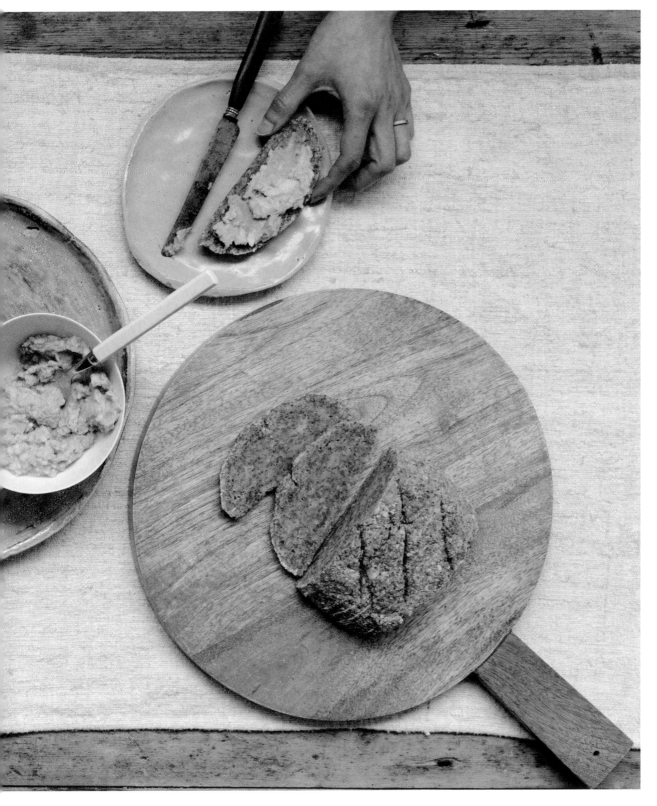

Grilled Portobello Mushrooms

This recipe is perfect for a weekend brunch when you fancy something savoury, filling and, of course, delicious. The mushrooms are a great base on which to pile the avocado and tomato filling, and they absorb the garlic and oil, which really helps to give the dish lots of flavour.

2 portobello mushrooms
1 garlic clove, crushed
2 tbsp olive oil,
    plus extra if needed
150g cherry tomatoes
1 avocado
½ lemon
salt and pepper

Preheat the grill.

Remove the stalks from your mushrooms and place to one side.

Combine the garlic with the olive oil in a small bowl. Then place the whole mushrooms into the bowl one by one and rub them with your fingers to coat them well. Place them under the grill for 12 minutes, turning halfway.

In the meantime, transfer any remaining garlic oil into a small saucepan and add a little more oil, if needed. Cut the tomatoes in half, then put these in with the oil and cook over a medium heat until soft, using the back of a wooden spoon to squash them slightly. You can add the mushroom stalks to avoid waste.

Halve the avocado, remove the stone and then mash the flesh well with a fork, adding salt, pepper and a squeeze of lemon.

Once the mushrooms are cooked, remove them from the grill, add the avocado and then spoon over the cooked tomatoes to serve.

02

light, fuss-free brunches

soups and salads

filling, fresh and simple

Pomegranate and Pistachio Salad

This is one of my favourite summer salads. It's bright, fresh and predominantly pink, with a creamy dressing that really brings out all of its wonderful flavours. It's a bit of a crowd pleaser and best enjoyed in a sunny garden.

I always used to buy pomegranate seeds that were ready to eat, which is pretty expensive. I then discovered a handy and, most importantly, mess-free way to deseed one myself, which has saved a lot of pink-splattered clothes and kitchen units. I have shared it in the method below – I hope you find it as revolutionary as I did.

For the salad
70g rocket
1 pomegranate
35g shelled pistachios
1 small raw beetroot
4 radishes, finely sliced
1 spring onion,
    finely sliced on
    the diagonal

For the dressing
juice of 1 lemon
2 tbsp tahini
2 tbsp olive oil
salt and pepper

Preheat the oven to 180°C/350°F/Gas Mark 4.

Divide the rocket leaves between two bowls.

Remove the seeds from the pomegranate. A great way to do this is by filling a bowl with cool water. This will stop you from getting covered in juice. Cut the pomegranate in half then submerge one half under water and ease the seeds out with your fingers. The pith will float and the seeds will sink, making it easier to separate them before draining. Repeat with the other half.

Place the pistachios on a baking tray and roast them for 5 minutes. Then remove, allow to cool and roughly chop.

Peel the beetroot and grate it using the regular side of a cheese grater.

Place all the salad ingredients in the bowls with the rocket.

Prepare the dressing by combining the lemon juice, tahini, olive oil, salt and pepper and mixing well.

Drizzle the dressing over the salad and toss well to combine.

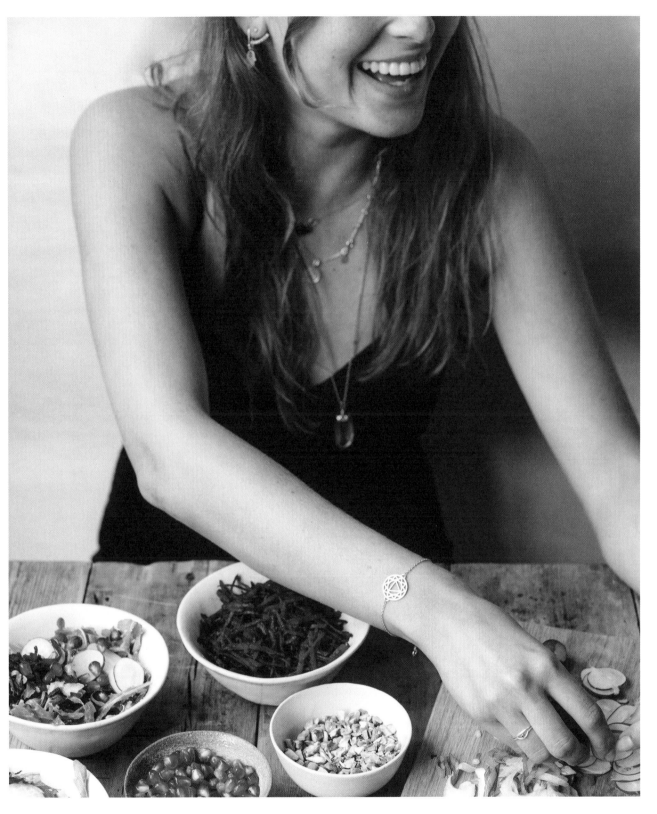

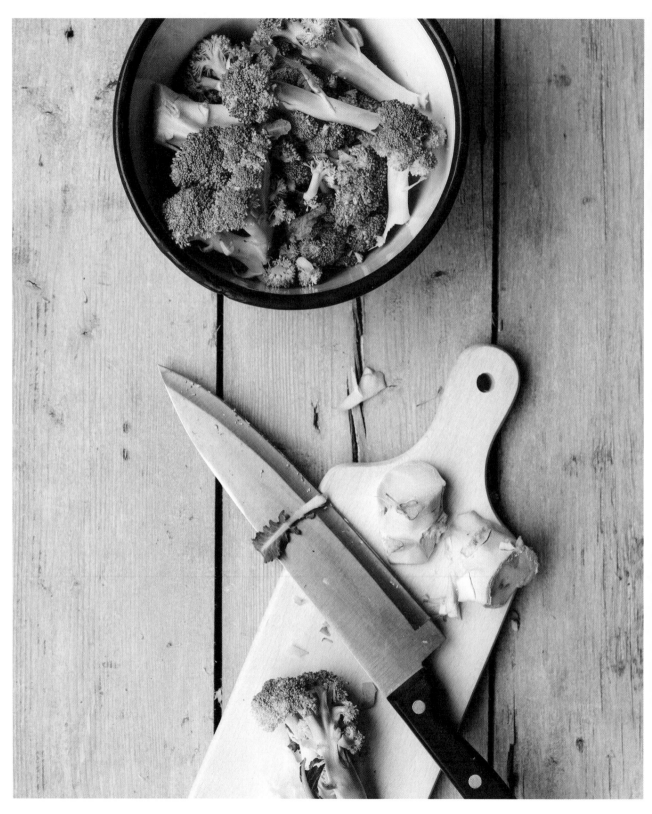

Pea and Broccoli Soup

Serves 2

This is a wonderfully clean-tasting soup, full of green goodness and flavour. The almond milk makes it thick and creamy, and it is remarkably filling and nutritious despite its simple ingredients list. The lemon really brings everything together and, depending on your palate, you can always add a little extra to give it a boost of freshness.

Start by boiling a full kettle.

Chop the broccoli into chunks, including the stem, then place in a steamer for 10 minutes or until soft.

Add the celery, miso paste and 700ml boiling water to a large saucepan, cover with a lid and simmer over a medium heat to make the stock while the broccoli cooks. After 20 minutes, add the peas and cook for 3 minutes.

Remove the broccoli from the steamer and transfer it to a blender, adding the garlic cloves, lemon juice and the pan of stock. Depending on the size of your blender, you may want to do this in batches. Blend well, adding the almond milk gradually until you have your desired consistency.

Pour the soup back into the pan over a medium heat to warm through before serving.

1 broccoli head
2 celery sticks, chopped
1 tbsp brown rice miso paste
300g frozen peas
2 garlic cloves
juice of 1 lemon
2 tbsp olive oil
200ml almond milk

Roasted Pepper and Buckwheat Salad

This wonderful salad is packed with simple but delicious Mediterranean-inspired flavours. It is full of colour, and the buckwheat gives it a filling quality that will leave you feeling light but satisfied.

2 garlic cloves, crushed
2 orange peppers,
 deseeded and cut
 into 2cm squares
2 red peppers,
 deseeded and cut
 into 2cm squares
1 tbsp olive oil
200g buckwheat groats
1 tsp tamari
juice of 1 lemon
100g pitted black
 olives, halved
100g rocket
salt and pepper

Preheat the oven to 180°C/350°F/Gas Mark 4.

Place the garlic in a roasting tin with the peppers and drizzle with the olive oil. Season with salt and pepper and roast for 40 minutes, mixing occasionally to cook evenly. Once they are starting to brown, remove them from the oven.

After 20–25 minutes, place the buckwheat groats in a pan with 375ml boiling water, the tamari and the juice from the lemon. Cook over a medium heat, stirring regularly, for 10–12 minutes until almost all the liquid has been absorbed from the buckwheat but it isn't totally dry. You can drain off any excess liquid if necessary.

Place the olives in a large serving bowl.

Once everything is done, add the buckwheat, peppers and any juices that are left in the roasting tin to the serving bowl. If you want to eat this dish warm, just mix in the rocket and serve straight away. Otherwise, leave everything until you want to serve before mixing in the leaves so that they don't wilt.

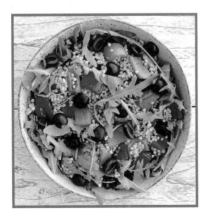

Gazpacho

This soup is based on a traditional gazpacho, although I came to it through impatience when I was too hungry to make my usual tomato soup.

At the time I was cooking for a friend and we both fancied something with a real kick, but the chilli is optional. I added a red pepper for sweetness and used cherry tomatoes, as they tend to be a little more sugary than regular ones. The cucumber helps to get the right consistency, thinning out the gazpacho with a refreshing flavour that you don't get with water. I really like a little bit of texture with my soup so I often serve it with a perfectly ripe avocado, which works like a dream, totally complementing the creamy soup while adding a little bite.

Add the tomatoes, red pepper, cucumber and cumin to a blender and whizz. If it struggles to get going, add 1–2 tablespoons water, although the cucumber and tomato juice should provide enough liquid for the soup to blend easily.

Add the chilli little by little until you get your spice level right and season with salt and pepper to taste.

Place the gazpacho in the fridge to cool if necessary.

Divide the avocado among the servings (if using), then add a sprig of basil and enjoy!

This soup lasts very well in the fridge for 3 days.

650g cherry tomatoes, roughly chopped
400g tomatoes, roughly chopped
1 red pepper, deseeded and roughly chopped
120g cucumber, roughly chopped
1 tsp ground cumin
1 fresh red chilli, deseeded and chopped
1 avocado, halved, pitted, skinned and finely sliced – optional
basil leaves, to garnish
salt and pepper

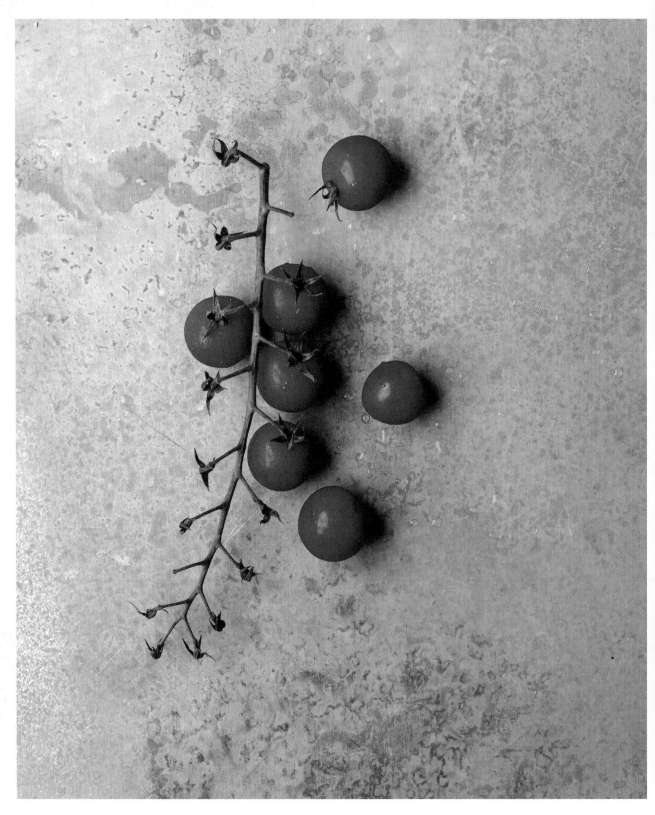

Soups and salads   184

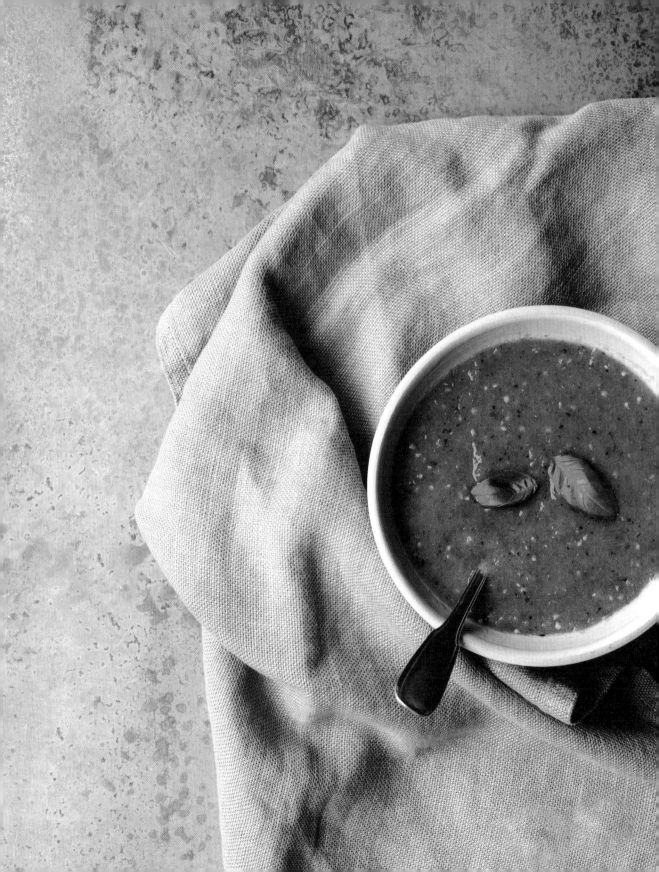

Turmeric, Carrot and Coconut Soup

I love this soup. It is so full of immune-boosting goodness and is perfect for days when you feel as though you are fighting something off. The ginger and chilli help to give it a bit of a kick, while the sweetness of the carrots and the coconut milk blend to make a delicious and smooth soup.

The cinnamon works perfectly with the coconut, and the chickpeas are ever so slightly sweet, too, adding both flavour and texture to your soup.

For the soup
2.5cm fresh ginger, peeled and finely chopped
½ fresh red chilli, deseeded and finely chopped
2 garlic cloves, finely chopped
1 tsp olive oil
1 heaped tsp ground turmeric
500g carrots, chopped
400ml tin coconut milk
1 tsp brown miso paste
salt and pepper

For the chickpeas
½ tsp ground cinnamon
1 tsp olive oil
400g tin chickpeas, drained and rinsed

Preheat the oven to 180°C/350°F/Gas Mark 4.

Add the ginger, chilli and garlic to a large pan with the olive oil and turmeric. Stir over a low heat until you can hear the spices start to sizzle, then add the carrots, coconut milk, miso paste and seasoning, as well as 200ml water. Cover with a lid and simmer for 20 minutes or until the carrots are completely soft.

To make the chickpeas, in a small bowl combine the cinnamon, oil and a little salt and pepper. Mix well, then add the drained chickpeas to evenly coat them in the oil. Transfer to a small roasting tin and bake for 15–20 minutes until crispy.

Once the carrots are soft, pour the contents of the pan into a blender and whizz until smooth.

Serve immediately, topped with the chickpeas, or keep some in the fridge – it's great cold, too!

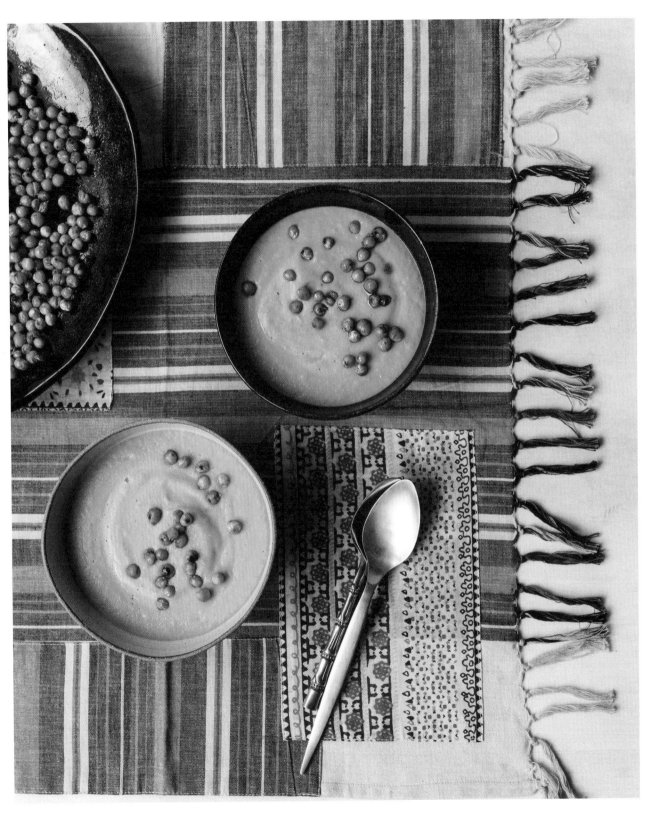

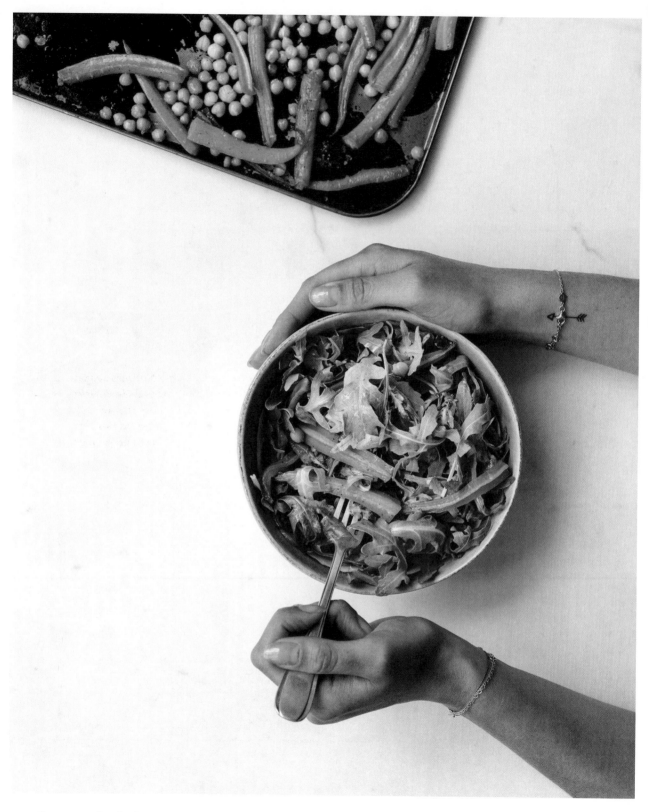

Honey-Roasted Carrot and Chickpea Salad

Simple salads don't have to be boring. I love that this one is fuss-free and has so few ingredients, yet it still tastes great. It's quite light, making it a great summer salad for when the weather is a bit warmer. The chickpeas give it a nice helping of plant protein, which helps to make it more filling than you'd expect. Sweet, peppery and citrussy – delicious!

Preheat the oven to 180°C/350°F/Gas Mark 4.

Place the carrots on a baking tray, and add the oil, honey and a generous sprinkle of salt and pepper. Mix well, then roast for 35 minutes.

Add the chickpeas to the baking tray, stir to mix with the carrots and cook for a further 10 minutes.

Once the chickpeas and carrots are ready, add them and the rocket to a serving bowl (you can serve the salad warm or wait for it to cool first). Mix everything together, adding the lemon juice before serving.

500g carrots, cut into batons
2 tbsp olive oil
1 tsp honey
400g tin chickpeas, drained and rinsed
70g rocket
juice of ½ lemon
salt and pepper

Kale and Raspberry Salad

Once I discovered how much I love the combination of tahini and raspberry, I couldn't get enough of it for a while – you may have already spotted it in the breakfast section! If you enjoyed that porridge, then hopefully you'll like this recipe, too. It's a spin on my favourite kale salad – I make some variation of it at least twice a week. I don't know if I will ever get sick of it!

100g kale, thick
    stalks removed
1 avocado, halved,
    pitted, skinned
    and diced
50g raspberries
a sprinkle of
    sesame seeds

For the dressing
125g raspberries
2 tbsp tahini
2 tbsp sesame oil
2 tsp tamari

Place the kale leaves in a large mixing bowl, ripping any large leaves into bite-sized pieces.

In a blender, whizz the ingredients for the dressing until you have a smooth consistency.

Pour the dressing over the kale and then use your hands to massage the dressing into the leaves so that they begin to soften.

Mix the avocado into the leaves. Serve the salad topped with the raspberries and sprinkled with sesame seeds.

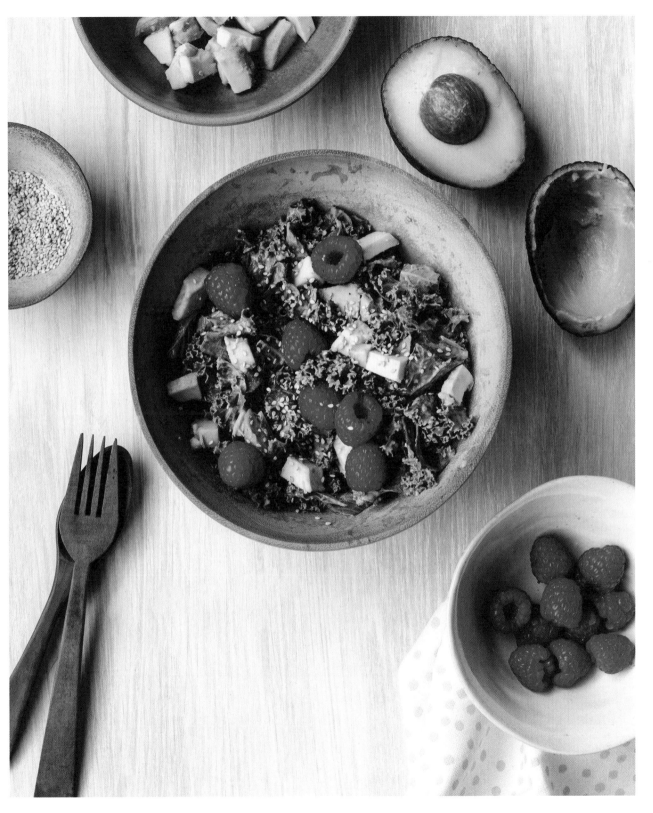

Sun-dried Tomato, Chickpea and Quinoa Salad

I love this salad. It is incredibly simple and uses just a few ingredients, most of which you probably already have in your cupboard at home. It takes only about 20 minutes to put together, so it makes a great dinner after a long day.

Tomato, basil, garlic and lemon combine to give the dish a real freshness. There is nothing fussy about it. I have added flaked almonds to give an extra crunch, and these also bring out the nutty flavour of the quinoa. The peas and sun-dried tomatoes give a gentle sweetness to the dish, while the black pepper balances out the overall flavour.

1½ lemons
180g quinoa
150g frozen peas
1 tbsp olive oil
2 large garlic cloves, crushed
400g tin chickpeas, drained and rinsed
100g flaked almonds
150g sun-dried tomatoes, finely chopped
50g basil leaves, finely chopped
salt and pepper

Boil a kettle of water – enough for two small pans.

Zest and juice 1 of the lemons, then cook the quinoa in boiling water according to the packet instructions – usually 1 part quinoa to 3 parts water is about right – adding the lemon juice. Keep an eye on the quinoa as it absorbs the water, making sure it doesn't dry out. It only takes 12–15 minutes to cook.

Boil the peas for just a few minutes until they are hot through but still firm. Then drain and place to one side.

In a large pan, heat the olive oil and garlic. Thoroughly coat the garlic in oil to prevent it from sticking, then add the chickpeas and flaked almonds, and stir well.

Once the chickpeas begin to heat through, after 2 minutes, add the quinoa, sun-dried tomatoes and the peas to the pan for a further 1–2 minutes until everything is hot.

Remove from the heat, add the chopped basil, lemon zest, lots of black pepper and a little salt to taste, squeezing over the last half of lemon. Give everything a good mix to serve.

03

colourful bowls and hearty meals

good for the body and soul

Red Rice Bowl with Beetroot Hummus

This dish was inspired by one of my favourite spots in Berlin, a small café tucked away on a back street in Mitte. Their menu is simple – a green bowl, a red bowl and a few others that I've never tried. I've visited twice and although I considered trying something different, I was drawn back to the red bowl that I loved so much the first time.

When I came to make this recipe at home I had to imagine what might be in it, as I never got round to asking, but I'm so happy with this version. I love the simplicity of this dish. It feels so nourishing with the contrasting textures, lots of raw veggies and tangy citrus dressing bringing it all together. The dressing is sharp, but if that's not your thing, you can tone down the lime or brown rice vinegar, or even sweeten it a little.

For the hummus
2 raw beetroots
juice of ½ lemon
1 tbsp tahini
400g tin chickpeas,
    drained and rinsed
4 tbsp olive oil, plus
    extra if needed
roughly chopped
    coriander leaves,
    to serve – optional
salt and pepper

Put the whole beetroots in a pan and cover generously with water. Bring to the boil, then simmer for 45 minutes. Turn off the heat and leave the beetroots to cool in the liquid. Drain. When cold, use your fingers to peel off the skin, then cut into dice.

Place the rice in a saucepan with 500ml boiling water. Cook for 30–35 minutes, or according to the packet instructions. You want the rice to be soft but still keeping its chewy texture. Drain.

Meanwhile, to make the dressing, place the lime juice in a small bowl with all the other dressing ingredients and stir well. Season with salt and pepper, and add extra maple syrup to sweeten it if you like.

(Continued on page 196.)

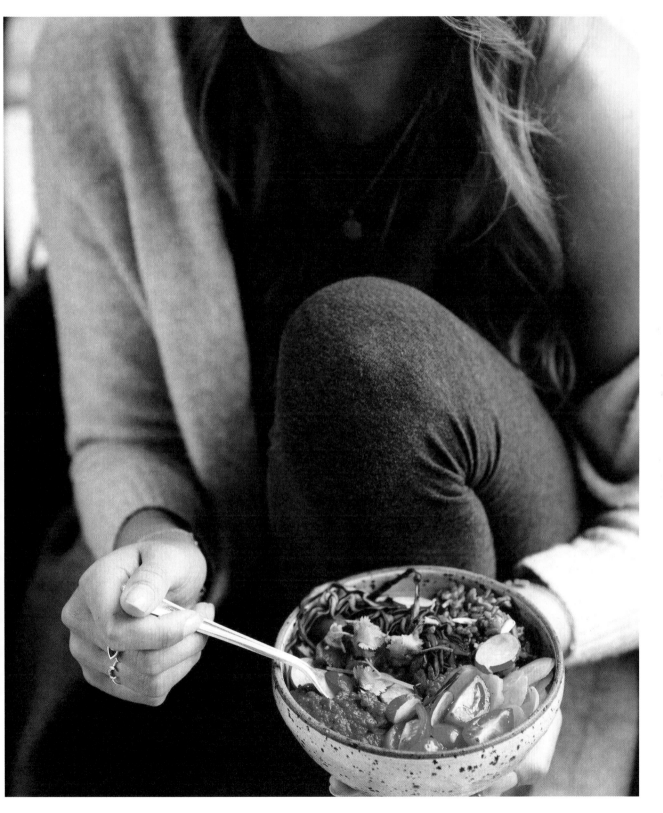

For the rice
120g red Camargue rice
2 tsp tahini
20g sunflower seeds

For the dressing
juice of 3 limes
3 tbsp brown
    rice vinegar
4 tbsp olive oil
3 tsp maple syrup,
    or to taste

For the salad
1 large carrot,
    thinly sliced
100g radishes,
    thinly sliced
200g red cabbage,
    cored and
    finely shredded
8 cherry tomatoes,
    quartered

Combine all the ingredients for the hummus, except the coriander, in a food processor. Blend until the hummus is smooth, seasoning with salt and pepper and adding a little more oil or water if needed, bit by bit.

Stir the tahini and sunflower seeds into the rice.

Once everything is prepared, place the salad veggies in a large bowl, then add the rice and hummus before drizzling with a generous amount of dressing and perhaps scattering over some coriander, to serve.

Creamy Aubergine and Asparagus Rice Bowl

This is a wonderfully comforting dish – the creamy texture really makes me feel warm and cosy. However, I love that it still remains fairly light compared to a heavy comfort-food meal. It is full of flavour and the dressing just lifts the whole dish. The pomegranate adds a fruitiness that works well with the asparagus to balance the bowl.

Preheat the oven to 180°C/350°F/Gas Mark 4.

Cook the rice according to the packet instructions. Make sure that the water doesn't completely evaporate. This should take 20–30 minutes.

Cut the aubergine in half lengthways. Using a small sharp knife, score the flesh in a crisscross pattern. Place on a baking tray.

In a small bowl mix together the maple syrup and miso paste to form a loose paste, then spread over the aubergine halves. Place the tray in the oven for 25 minutes.

Prepare the dressing by placing all the ingredients in a small bowl and stirring well.

Add the garlic to a frying pan over a medium–low heat with the olive oil and onion. Once the onion is almost totally translucent, add the asparagus. Stir regularly to prevent anything from burning. Once the asparagus is soft but still has bite to it, turn off the heat. This takes about 7 minutes.

When the aubergine has softened, remove it from the oven and place it in a food processor with the tahini. Whizz for a few seconds so that it breaks down but isn't totally smooth. Then scoop it out and place it in the pan with the onion and asparagus, stirring in the rice until everything is evenly mixed.

Drizzle over the dressing and mix through before sprinkling the pomegranate seeds on top to serve.

180g short-grain brown rice
1 aubergine
1 tbsp maple syrup
1 tbsp brown rice miso paste
2 garlic cloves, crushed
1 tbsp olive oil
1 onion, chopped
200g asparagus, cut into 1cm long pieces
1 tbsp tahini
75g pomegranate seeds

For the dressing
1 tbsp tahini
1 tsp brown rice miso paste
2 tbsp sesame oil
1 tbsp maple syrup
juice of ½ lemon
¼ fresh red chilli, deseeded and finely chopped – optional

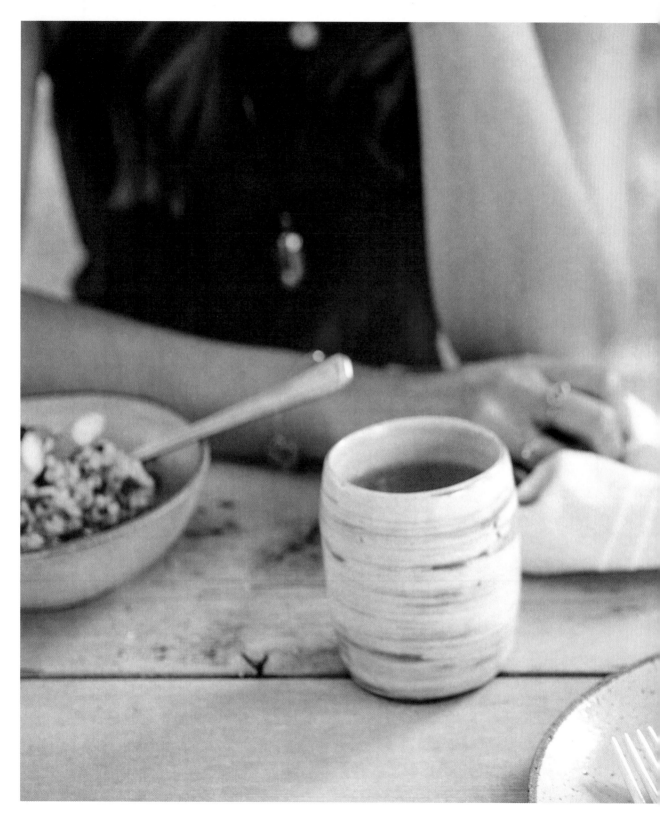

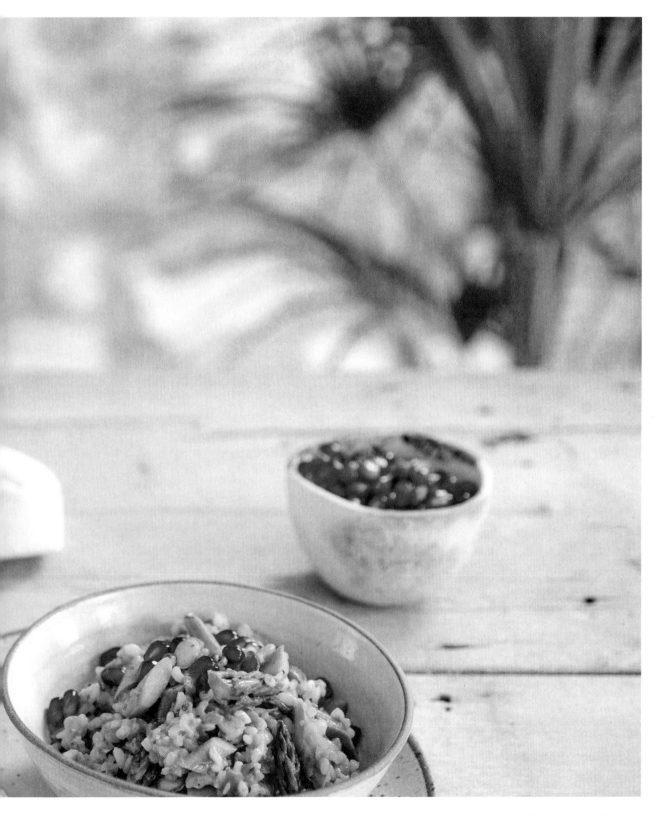

Simple Ratatouille

This recipe reminds me of my dad. He is the ratatouille king and so I had him try this one out to see how it compared to his own. When my sister and I were growing up I remember complaining that he gave us ratatouille that was a day old (we had a period of time where we were terrified of getting sick from leftover food, despite it never having happened to either of us). He assured us that it got better each day it was left in the fridge, and he couldn't be more right. The flavour becomes richer the longer you leave this dish, and so I always make a huge batch and eat it over the course of the week, adding it to salads, rice bowls or whatever else I might be having.

1 aubergine, cut into
   2cm squares
1 courgette, cut into
   2cm squares
2 red peppers,
   deseeded and cut
   into 2cm squares
4 garlic cloves, crushed
2 tbsp olive oil
2 red onions, chopped
1 tsp dried mixed
   herbs (I like herbes
   de Provence)
8 tomatoes,
   roughly chopped
2 tbsp tomato purée
salt and pepper

Place the aubergine, courgette and red peppers in a large saucepan over a medium-low heat and cover with a lid, allowing them to sweat for 8 minutes. Remove from the pan and set aside.

Add the garlic to a large pan with the olive oil and gently heat for 1–2 minutes, then add the onions, allowing them to soften for 5 minutes.

Return the aubergine, courgette, red peppers and mixed herbs to the pan, adding a generous amount of pepper and some salt before stirring well to coat the vegetables. After 5 minutes, add the tomatoes and tomato purée and then cover the pan with a lid to cook for 25 minutes or until softened.

Remove the lid and allow a little liquid to boil off – I do this for about 3 minutes. Once the vegetables are soft but not totally mushy, remove the ratatouille from the heat to serve, seasoning well with more salt and pepper if needed.

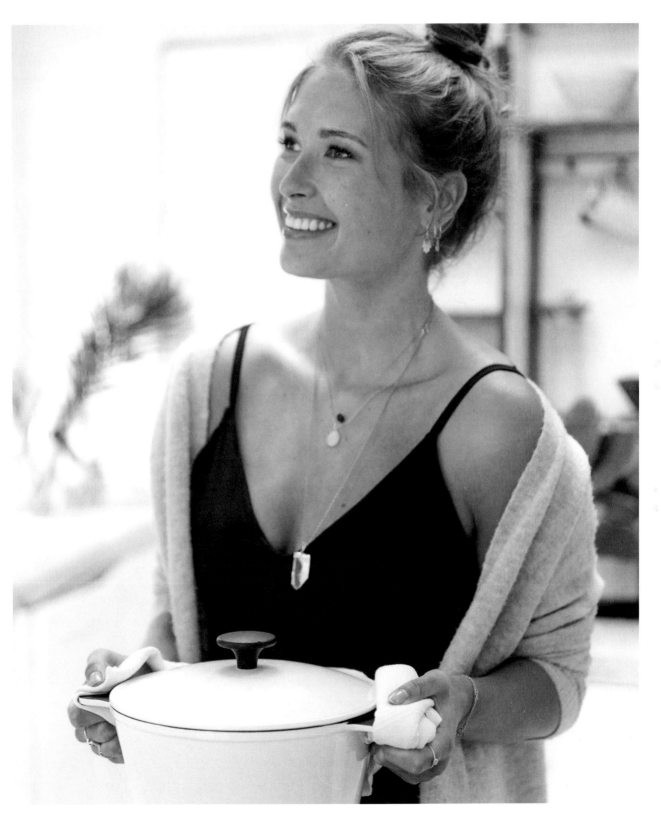

Mexican Bowl

I love how bright this bowl is – it's full of colour, flavour and textures that work together perfectly. Each of the four elements is absolutely delicious in its own right, too: sweet potato fries, brown rice, black beans and a guacamole all served on little gem lettuce to add extra greenery and crunch.

1 little gem lettuce
a small handful of
    coriander, leaves
    chopped, to serve
    – optional
salt and pepper
extra lime juice, to serve

For the sweet potato
    curly fries
1 sweet potato
3 tbsp olive oil
3 tbsp buckwheat flour
2 tsp paprika

For the rice
100g short-grain
    brown rice
1 tsp brown rice
    miso paste

For the guacamole
1 avocado
juice of ½ lime
5g coriander leaves,
    finely chopped
8 cherry tomatoes,
    quartered
¼–½ fresh red chilli,
    to taste, deseeded,
    if you like, and
    finely chopped
salt and pepper

Preheat the oven to 180°C/350°F/Gas Mark 4.

Start with the sweet potatoes. Spiralize the sweet potato if you have a spiralizer to make curly fries. If not, you can always make these into wedges and allow them a little longer to cook.

Place the curly fries or wedges in a large baking dish, and cover with the oil, flour and paprika. Season with salt and pepper, and mix well (I use my hands).

Place in the oven for 30 minutes until crisp, checking regularly and mixing so that they cook evenly.

While the sweet potato cooks, start on the rice. Boil the rice in a pan with the miso paste and 200ml boiling water, adding more water as necessary. I like the rice to keep a bit of bite to it, but you can cook it to your desired texture, of course. It should take 20–30 minutes.

For the guacamole, halve, pit and skin the avocado, then mash it in a bowl with the lime juice. Mix all the ingredients together, adding the chilli last and gradually until it's the right heat for you.

Prop up a few lettuce leaves in each of the two bowls.

When the rice and sweet potatoes are almost cooked, gently heat the black beans in a small pan with the cayenne pepper and tomato purée. Add the lime zest and juice to the pan.

Add each component to the bowls of lettuce to serve, along with a sprinkling of chopped coriander, if you like, and a squeeze of extra lime juice to taste, and season with salt and pepper.

For the black beans
400g tin black beans, drained and rinsed
¼ tsp cayenne pepper
2 tsp tomato purée
zest of 1 lime and juice of ½ lime

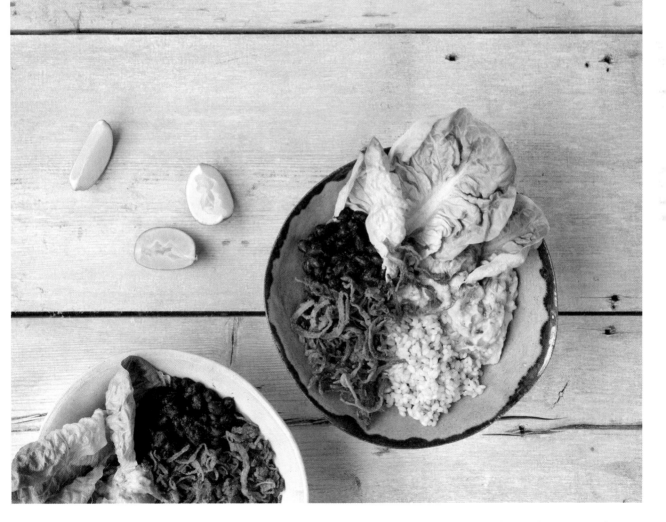

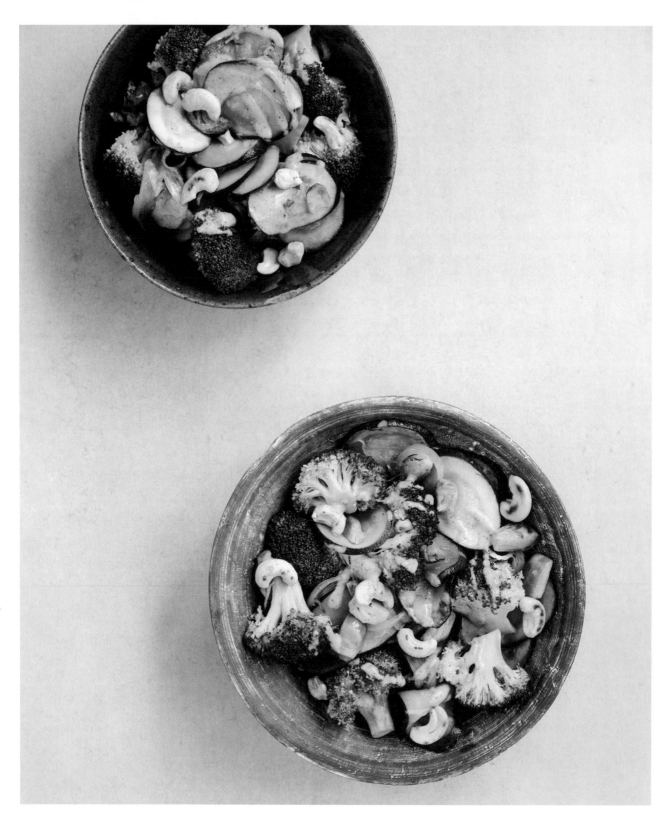

Green Goddess Bowl

This is a great meal for when you're craving something nourishing and comforting but don't fancy the heaviness of grains or beans. Vegetable-based, it'll leave you feeling light and virtuous while the almond butter dressing keeps you full. If you're looking for a real boost of green, I hope this gives you the hit you need!

Angle the knife and finely chop the courgettes into diagonal slices.

Toast the cashews in a dry pan over a low heat until lightly golden. Remove from the pan and put to one side.

In a large frying pan, over a medium–high heat, fry the onion in the olive oil with the salt. Once it has softened, remove from the pan and add the broccoli and Brussels sprouts, and fry for 7 minutes, until they are dark green but still have a bite. Remove these from the pan and leave to one side.

Add the courgette and the tamari to the pan and fry for 5 minutes, until brown on each side and slightly softened. Add the broccoli, onion and sprouts back in the pan to warm through while you make the dressing.

In a small bowl, combine all the dressing ingredients. Add 45ml water gradually until you get your desired consistency. Drizzle over the cooked vegetables and scatter over the toasted cashews to serve.

400g courgettes
60g cashews
1 small onion, finely sliced
1 tbsp olive oil
a pinch of salt
1 broccoli head (you can throw the stalk in, too), cut into bite-sized pieces
200g Brussels sprouts, quartered
2 tsp tamari

For the dressing
juice of 1 lemon
2 tbsp almond butter
2 tbsp olive oil

Mushroom Quinoa Burger with Black Bean Sauce

When people hear that I don't eat meat, they often ask, 'But don't you ever just want a juicy burger?' For me, the honest answer is never. I can appreciate the look of a good burger, but I have never once thought about eating one. It just wouldn't do it for me. That said, I do enjoy veggie 'burgers' – you can blend so many different ingredients for a delicious alternative.

This burger is best served on a bed of sautéed spinach, and you can even add a side of spiralized sweet potato (page 202) and a few slices of lightly toasted bread for a healthy spin on the traditional burger and chips comfort-food combo.

150g quinoa
1 tsp brown rice
    miso paste
1 red onion, chopped
2 tbsp olive oil,
    plus extra for frying
2 garlic cloves, crushed
150g mushrooms,
    finely chopped
50g buckwheat or
    brown rice flour
1 heaped tsp paprika
2 tsp apple cider vinegar
salt and pepper

Start by cooking the quinoa in boiling water according to the instructions on the packet – usually 1 part quinoa to 3 parts water is about right. Add the miso paste and stir well. Keep an eye on the quinoa as it absorbs the water, making sure it doesn't dry out too quickly. It takes 12–15 minutes to cook so in the meantime prepare the veg.

Add the onion to a frying pan with the 2 tablespoons olive oil and then add the garlic. Fry over a medium heat, stirring regularly to prevent it from burning. Add the mushrooms as the onion turns translucent. Fry for 5 minutes or until the mushrooms have become golden brown.

Once the quinoa is cooked, drain off any excess water and put it in a large mixing bowl with the onion and mushrooms. Mix in the flour, paprika and apple cider vinegar, mixing well and seasoning with salt and pepper. Set this to one side to cool.

Place all the black bean sauce ingredients in a food processor with 75ml water and mix until it makes a smooth, thick sauce. Then transfer it into a saucepan to heat through.

In your frying pan, heat a glug of olive oil for shallow frying over a medium heat. Take a large handful of the quinoa burger mix and squash it firmly between your hands – it can help if your hands are slightly wet. Put it into the pan and press down firmly with a spatula. Repeat three more times so that you have four large burgers, or until you have used up all the mixture.

When the burgers begin to brown on one side, after 4 minutes, flip them over, pressing them down again. Once the burgers have browned on both sides, about 7 minutes in total, they are ready. Pour over the black bean sauce to serve.

For the black bean sauce
400g tin black beans, drained and rinsed
2 tsp tomato purée
4 tbsp brown rice vinegar
1 tbsp maple syrup
2 tsp tamari

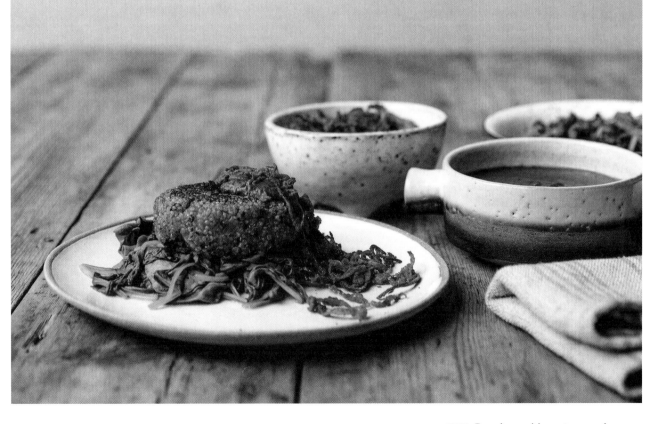

Raw Courgetti with Sun-dried Tomato Pesto and Cashew Cream

This is a wonderful dish, perfect for a summer's day or when you are looking for something light but still delicious. It can be served raw or warmed through to suit your mood, too.

4 courgettes
75g sunflower seeds
   – optional

For the cashew cream
100g cashews
1–2 garlic cloves
juice of ½ lemon
4g nutritional yeast
salt and pepper

For the pesto
1 broccoli head
150g sun-dried tomatoes
juice of ½ lemon
45ml olive oil (you may
   choose to add
   a little more if your
   tomatoes didn't
   come in oil)

Use a spiralizer to make the courgetti. You can also use a julienne peeler or a vegetable peeler to make thin strips instead.

Place all the ingredients for the cashew cream into a blender and add up to 60ml water, bit by bit. You may not need all the water and you might need to use a spatula to make sure all the mixture is blended. I prefer to keep it a little bit chunky, but you can keep blending until smooth if you prefer. Scoop it all out and leave to one side.

Roughly chop the broccoli head and add it to the cleaned blender, along with the sun-dried tomatoes, lemon juice and oil, then add up to 100ml water little by little until everything is broken down and evenly blended. Again, you may want a little more or less water, so add it gradually, seasoning to taste.

In a large mixing bowl combine the courgette noodles and pesto and mix well – I usually use my hands to make sure it is evenly covered. Serve with the cashew cream and sprinkle with sunflower seeds, if desired.

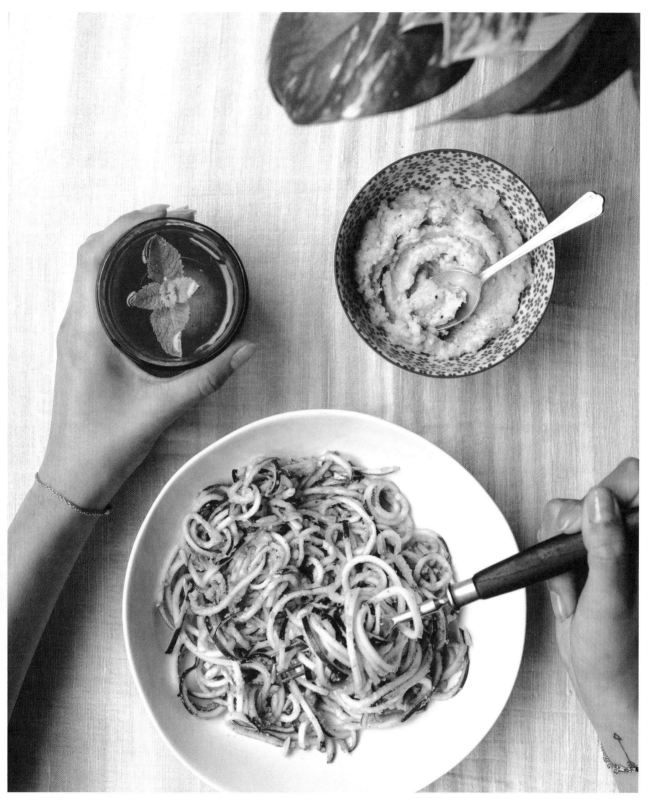

Baked Sweet Potato with Lentil Dhal

This is a really comforting and filling dish, perfect for a winter evening or when you are looking for something simple but substantial. The sweetness of the potatoes is complemented perfectly by the slight spice of the dhal, bringing together a wonderfully hearty and wholesome dish.

3 sweet potatoes
140g red lentils
1 tsp brown rice
    miso paste
1 tbsp olive oil
1 tsp cumin seeds
3cm fresh ginger, peeled
    and finely chopped
½–1 tsp chilli powder,
    to taste
1 bay leaf
1 onion, finely chopped
3 garlic cloves, crushed
300g cherry tomatoes,
    chopped
a few handfuls of
    mixed leaves,
    (rocket, spinach,
    etc.) – optional
salt and pepper

Preheat the oven to 180°C/350°F/Gas Mark 4.

Use a fork to prick the potatoes all over and then place them on a baking tray in the oven for 45 minutes–1 hour (depending on the size).

Rinse the lentils, then cover with 600ml boiling water and allow to boil. Reduce the heat, removing any froth and adding the brown miso paste, and simmer for 25 minutes, adding extra water if needed, until the lentils are soft. Drain any remaining water.

In a large pan, heat the olive oil and the cumin seeds. When the seeds start to jump, add the ginger, chilli powder, bay leaf, onion and garlic. Keep the heat medium–low and let the onion soften slowly.

Add the cherry tomatoes to the pan once the onion has softened, using the back of a wooden spoon to squash them. Season with salt and pepper.

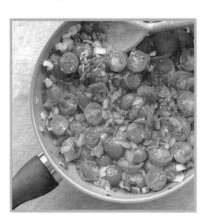

Turn off the heat and place to one side until the lentils and the potatoes are ready, then add the lentils to the tomato mixture, stirring to incorporate, and heat through. Season to taste and remove and discard the bay leaf.

Cut the potatoes lengthways and add the dhal, serving with a handful of mixed leaves, if you like.

Rainbow Buddha Bowl with Sweet Potato Hummus

Serves 2

This bowl is so full of colour, it really does help you to eat the rainbow. I love the sweet potato hummus and it works wonderfully as a stand-alone dish, too. The quinoa and chickpeas provide a good dose of plant protein and everything is pulled together by a fresh miso dressing, giving you a great-tasting, colourful meal to fuel you up with long-lasting energy.

To make the hummus, place the sweet potato chunks in a steamer and cook for 10–15 minutes or until they are soft all the way through.

In the meantime, cook the quinoa according to the packet instructions, adding the juice of ½ lemon and the tamari to the water for flavour.

Peel the beetroot and grate it using the coarse side of a grater, and then add to the serving bowls.

Mix all the dressing ingredients together in a small bowl, ready to pour over at the end.

Once the sweet potato is soft, place in a food processor with the garlic, tahini, chickpeas, olive oil, salt and cumin until a smooth hummus forms.

When the quinoa is cooked, spoon it into your bowls. Add the rocket and sweet potato hummus, then top with radishes and spring onions, and drizzle over the miso dressing. You can use the remaining lemon to squeeze over to your taste.

100g quinoa
juice of 1 lemon
1 tsp tamari
1 raw beetroot
30g rocket
70g radishes,
    finely sliced
2 spring onions,
    finely sliced

For the hummus
1 small sweet potato,
    cut into small chunks
1 garlic clove
1 tsp tahini
½ x 400g tin chickpeas,
    drained and rinsed
3 tbsp olive oil
a large pinch of salt
½ tsp ground cumin

For the dressing
1 tsp brown rice
    miso paste
2 tbsp olive oil
½ lemon

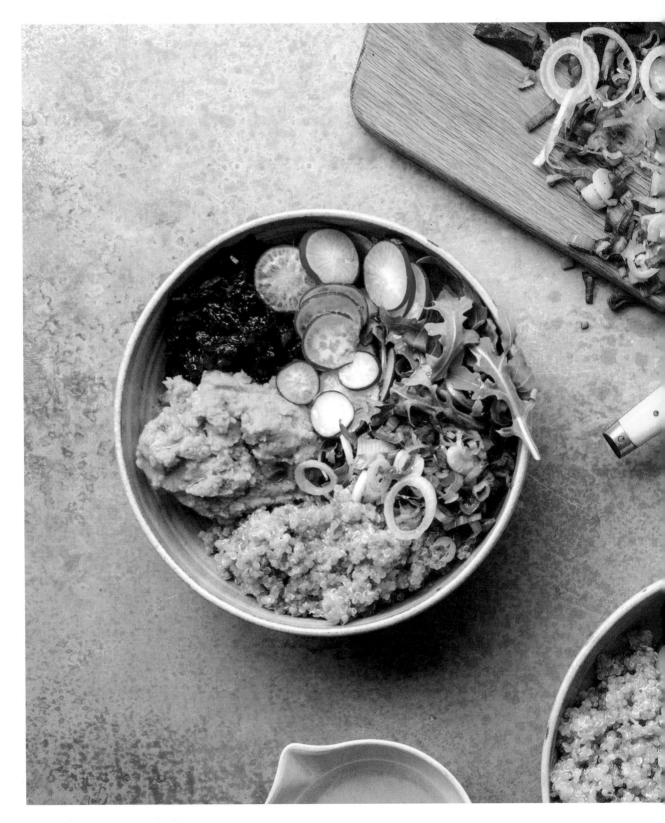

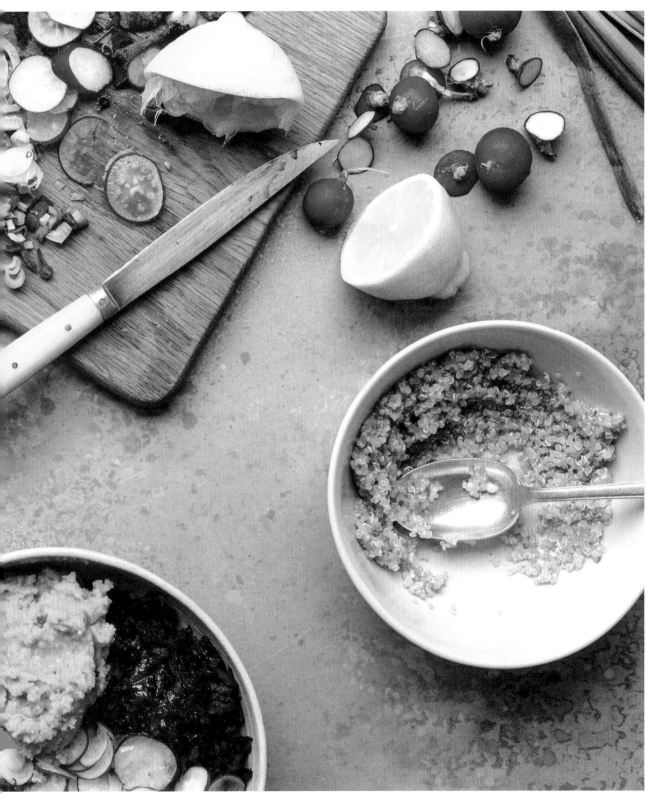

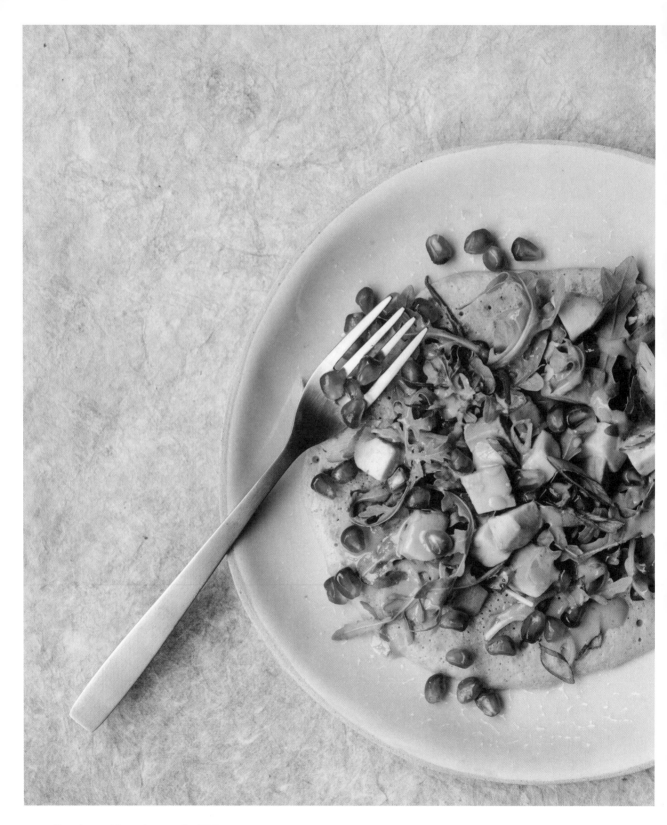

Middle Eastern Pancake with Pomegranate and Avocado

I think this could be one of my favourite recipes in the book, and the funny thing is that it came about by accident. I had a fridge full of ingredients ready for various meals I'd planned, but ended up making this instead. I love impromptu recipes, especially when they taste this good. It looks kind of fancy, too, so it's great for showing off without too much effort.

Sift the flour into a large mixing bowl, then add the remaining pancake ingredients except the coconut oil. Season with salt and pepper and add 175ml water. Whisk it well to combine thoroughly and set aside for 10–30 minutes (the longer the better, but if you're in a hurry it will still work fine).

While you wait, you can make the dressing. Simply combine the tahini, tamari and sesame oil in a small bowl and stir well, then add 1–2 tablespoons water gradually until you have a thick dressing.

Melt the coconut oil in a non-stick frying pan over a medium–high heat. Add some of the pancake batter to the pan, thicker than a crêpe, thinner than an American-style pancake. Gently heat it through for 2 minutes or until it is cooked on one side, then flip it over and let the other side cook for a further 2 minutes.

You can keep the pancakes warm in the oven on a low heat while you repeat with the remaining mixture.

Once cooked, top with the rocket, avocado chunks, spring onions and pomegranate seeds, drizzling over the dressing to serve.

For the pancake
120g gram flour
1 tsp ground cumin
2 tbsp olive oil
1 garlic clove,
    finely chopped
1 tsp coconut oil
salt and pepper

For the dressing
1 tbsp tahini
2 tsp tamari
1 tbsp sesame oil

For the topping
30g rocket
1 avocado, halved,
    pitted, skinned
    and cut into chunks
2 spring onions, finely
    sliced on the diagonal
50g pomegranate seeds
    (see method page 178)

Chickpea Curry

While I was in Goa, my absolute favourite dish was chana masala – a delicious chickpea curry – and I ate it almost every time I went out to eat. The way it was cooked, like much of the food there, was with a lot of oil, and, of course, a little spice. I wanted to recreate it at home, but with a slightly healthier twist by holding back on the oiliness, and while this does make a difference to the dish, it is just as delicious and still full of nostalgia for me.

75g brown rice
2 tbsp olive oil
2 large garlic
    cloves, crushed
2 tsp ground cumin
1 tsp ground turmeric
1 tsp garam masala
1 onion, finely chopped
1 fresh red chilli,
    deseeded and
    finely chopped
1cm piece of fresh
    ginger, peeled and
    finely chopped
125g cherry
    tomatoes, halved
400g tin chopped
    tomatoes or 200g
    of fresh tomatoes
400g tin chickpeas,
    drained and rinsed
100g spinach
juice of ½ lemon
a handful of coriander
    leaves chopped

Cook the rice according to the packet instructions. Usually a ratio of 2 parts water, 1 part rice is about right. Make sure that the water doesn't completely evaporate as you cook. This should take 20–30 minutes.

In a large saucepan, add the olive oil over a medium heat, then add the garlic and spices, and stir well.

Place the onion, chilli and ginger in the pan and allow the onion to soften, taking care not to let anything burn.

Once the onion has softened, add the cherry tomatoes and fresh tomatoes, if you are using those, halving or quartering them if you've chosen big ones. If you are using tinned tomatoes, wait until the cherry tomatoes have softened, then add these, the chickpeas and the spinach. Keep cooking until any watery liquid boils off and the curry thickens. Then squeeze in the lemon, stirring well before serving with the rice and garnishing with the chopped coriander.

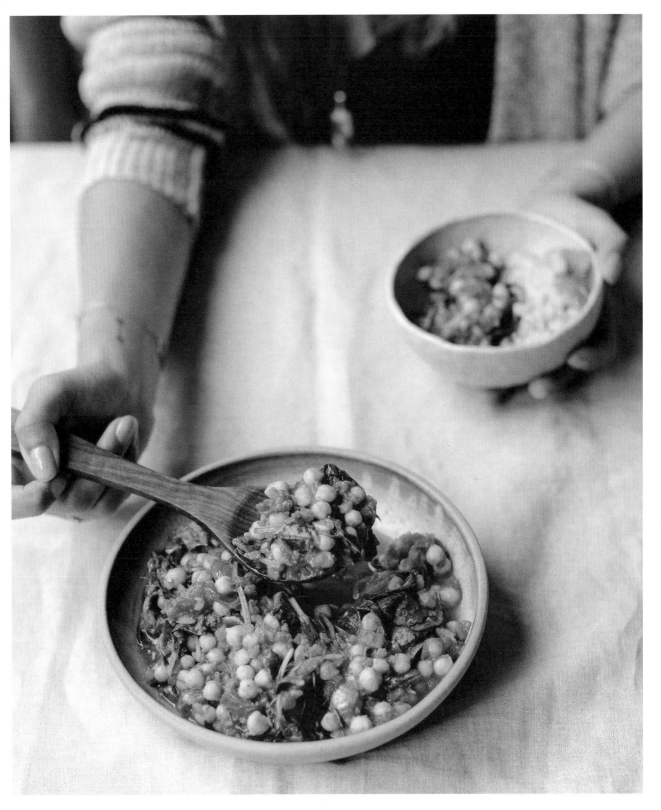

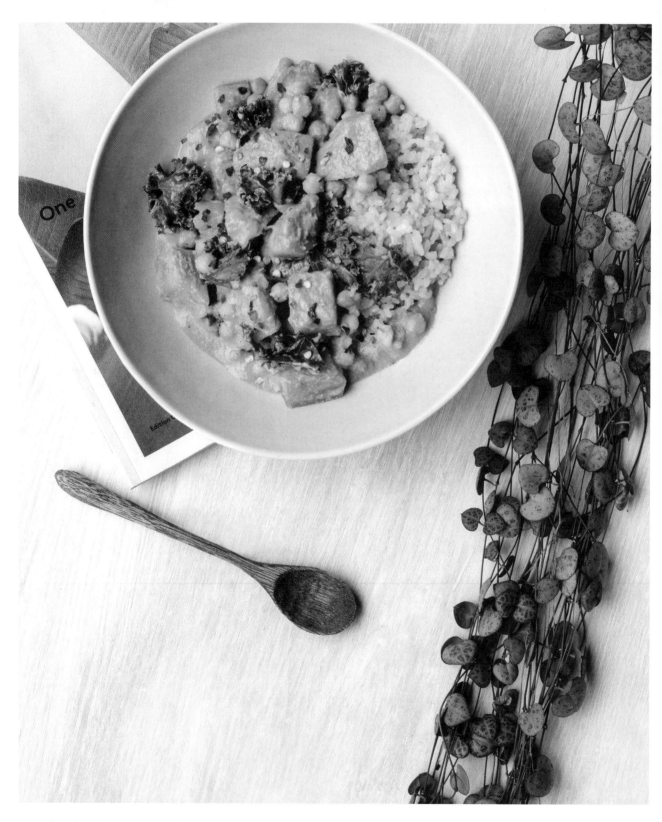

One

Edition

Butternut Squash and Kale Curry

I originally made this recipe when I was asked by a charity to produce an autumnal dish using seasonal ingredients. Since then it's been a favourite, and one I often make when I'm entertaining friends. The recipe includes a curry paste, which I use a lot at home, so it's a good staple to have if you like experimenting with curries. I sometimes serve this with brown rice, but it's great without and I usually find it filling enough on its own.

Cook the rice according to the packet instructions. Make sure that the water doesn't completely evaporate as you cook. This should take 20–30 minutes.

Next, make the curry paste. Place the paste ingredients in a blender and whizz until a paste forms.

Chop the creamed coconut and dissolve in 800ml boiling water to make coconut milk. Peel the butternut squash and cut into bite-sized chunks.

Add the curry paste to a large pan over a low heat and cook for 3 minutes, making sure it doesn't burn. Then add the coconut milk and stir thoroughly, bringing it to a boil. Add the butternut squash and lemongrass and cover with a lid. Turn the heat down and allow it to simmer for 10 minutes. Add the chickpeas and simmer for another 20 minutes until the squash starts to soften.

Remove the lid from the saucepan and add the lemon juice. Next, add the kale, allowing it to wilt for 5 minutes. Once the squash is soft, it is ready to serve. Remove the lemongrass stalk and discard, and then add a sprinkle of chilli flakes to taste.

200g short-grain brown rice
200g creamed coconut
1 butternut squash
1 lemongrass stalk
400g tin chickpeas, drained and rinsed
juice of 1 lemon
100g kale, tough stalks removed
chilli flakes, to taste

For the paste
1 shallot, chopped
3cm fresh ginger, peeled and chopped
4 garlic cloves, chopped
juice of 1 lime
2 tsp ground turmeric
2 tsp ground cumin
¼ tsp grated nutmeg
1 tsp ground cinnamon
¼ tsp ground cardamom
4 tbsp tamari
½ tbsp ground black pepper

Pea and Spinach Risotto

I have such a thing for pea and spinach as a flavour pairing.
I really find myself looking for any opportunity to include this
wonder combination in my life most days. This warming dish
is perfectly creamy and comforting, but it doesn't leave you
feeling overly full and heavy.

Brown rice, peas and spinach are all such awesome
ingredients, providing us with protein, fibre and a whole array
of vitamins and nutrients. Brown rice is a great swap for regular
risotto rice, keeping you fuller for longer and preventing energy
crashes after eating.

1 onion, finely chopped
2 tsp ground cumin
2 garlic cloves, crushed
2 tsp olive oil
260g short-grain
    brown rice
2 tsp sumac
300g peas
3 large handfuls
    of spinach
2 tbsp tahini
juice of 1 lime
salt and pepper

Place the onion in a large pan with the cumin, garlic, salt, pepper
and olive oil. Gently stir over a medium heat until the onion
becomes nicely covered and starts to soften.

Add the rice and stir thoroughly for 1 minute. Then add the sumac
and 600ml water, and bring to the boil.

Once the water is boiling, reduce the heat and leave to simmer for
10 minutes. Then add the peas and spinach and let it simmer again,
stirring occasionally until the water evaporates and the rice is soft
but still has a little bite to it. Mix in the tahini and the lime juice
and serve.

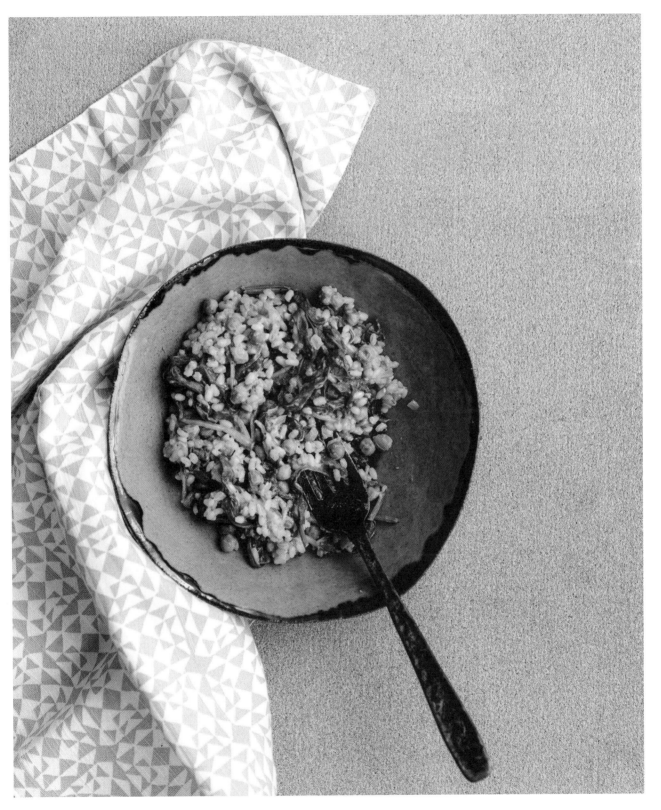

Creamy Mac and 'Cheese'

This dish is the ultimate comfort food. It takes me right back to winter evenings after school, when we would beg my mum to make us macaroni cheese, then fight over the crispy bits!

This is a healthier spin on an old favourite, inspired by the creamy comfort of cheese sauce but a little more green. I like to add veggies and love the sweetness of the peas, but you can leave them out if you fancy something a bit more familiar. This really is a great one for a lazy evening in and makes a generous amount so there's plenty to go around.

1 broccoli head, cut into small pieces
2 tbsp olive oil
200g brown rice penne pasta (or pasta of choice)
200g mushrooms, finely chopped
175g frozen peas

For the sauce
100g cashews
2 small potatoes, finely chopped
3 carrots, finely chopped
75ml almond milk or oat milk
1 tsp paprika
1 tsp ground cumin
juice of ¼ lemon
1 garlic clove
1 tbsp tamari
30g nutritional yeast, plus 5g to sprinkle on top
1 tbsp olive oil
salt and pepper

To make the sauce, soak the cashews in water for at least 1–1½ hours, or longer is even better, as this helps to soften them, making them blend more easily.

Preheat the oven to 180°C/350°F/Gas Mark 4 and boil a kettle.

Place the potatoes and carrots in a steamer. Steam for 35 minutes or until completely soft.

Drizzle the broccoli with 1 tablespoon of the olive oil and place in the oven to roast for 20 minutes or until soft.

Cook the pasta in boiling water according to the packet instructions, as the timings can vary from brand to brand.

Fry the mushrooms in a pan with the remaining oil over a medium heat for 10 minutes or until golden brown.

About 2 minutes before the pasta is done, add the peas to the pan to heat through. Make sure not to overcook the pasta. When it is done, take it off the heat, drain well and place in a mixing bowl, before adding the mushrooms.

Remove the broccoli from the oven and add to the mixing bowl.

Drain the cashews and remove the carrots and potato from the steamer once soft, placing them all in a blender with the other sauce ingredients. Blend well until smooth and season to taste with salt and pepper. Add to the mixing bowl and mix until everything is covered in the sauce.

You can stop here and choose to eat this as a creamy pasta dish, or pour it into a baking dish, topping with the remaining nutritional yeast and then baking for 15 minutes or until the top turns crispy.

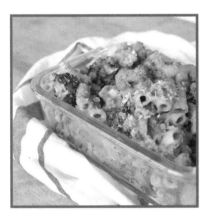

Lemon Chickpea Stew

This dish was inspired by a friend of mine who usually makes something similar with chicken. I've never tried the one she makes (being veggie), but I so loved the idea (and smell) of it that I decided to give it a try myself and see what I could come up with. I love the leeks in this dish – I tend to forget about them when I am experimenting with new recipes, but they work really well in this. You can always swap them for onion if they aren't your thing.

2 tsp brown rice
    miso paste
2 tbsp olive oil
2 garlic cloves, crushed
1 tsp cumin seeds
2 leeks, cut lengthways
    and sliced
2 × 400g tins chickpeas,
    drained and rinsed
zest and juice of
    2 lemons, plus
    wedges to serve
    – optional
300g frozen peas
4 tbsp coriander,
    roughly chopped
salt and pepper

Make the stock by dissolving the miso paste in 500ml boiling water.

In a large pan, heat the olive oil over a medium heat. Add the garlic with the cumin and the leeks to the pan. Stir well for 10 minutes or until the leek softens.

Add the chickpeas to the pan, and pour in the miso stock. Add two-thirds of the lemon juice to the pan. Let the liquid simmer for 20 minutes or until it begins to thicken, as the chickpeas will absorb the water. Before all the water disappears, add the peas and mix well to allow them to heat through.

Once the water has absorbed or boiled off almost completely and the chickpeas are nice and soft, remove the stew from the heat.

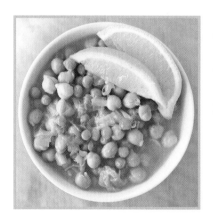

Stir the coriander through with the lemon zest before serving. Season with salt and pepper, add the remaining lemon juice to taste and serve with lemon wedges, if you like.

04

easy
versatile
sides
the perfect
match

Aubergine Dip

This aubergine dip is the perfect side dish to serve with any Middle Eastern or Mediterranean-style meal. It also makes an easy snack served on a rice cake or with crudités. It's pretty fuss-free but has a wonderfully creamy texture. I like to keep the seasoning simple, with just a little lemon, salt and pepper, so you don't have to worry about stocking up on lots of herbs and spices.

1 aubergine, halved lengthways
1 tbsp tahini
1 garlic clove
juice of ½ lemon
salt and pepper

Use a knife to score the flesh of the aubergine diagonally one way and then back the other way in a crisscross pattern.

Place a large non-stick pan over a medium-high heat and add the aubergine halves, flesh-side down, for 5 minutes, then flip and cook skin-side down for 12 minutes or until the flesh starts to burst out of the cuts and it becomes visibly soft. You will notice that it will start to collapse in on itself when it's ready.

Scoop out the soft flesh and put it in a food processor with the tahini and garlic. Blend everything together and season to taste with salt and pepper. Add the lemon bit by bit. I like adding it all, but you can use less if you like it less tart.

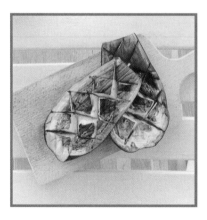

Potato Hash

This simple potato dish is a great tapas-style side, or even works as a savoury breakfast option on a lazy morning. The tomatoes and red pepper add a little sweetness, and the basil, garlic and red onion add some wonderful flavours.

In a large pan, heat the oil over a medium heat. Add the onion and garlic and allow to simmer gently for a few minutes until the onions begin to soften.

Add the potatoes to the pan and cover. Cook for 20 minutes or until the potatoes begin to soften, then add the tomatoes and red pepper. Cook for a further 10 minutes with the lid off, using the back of a spoon to mash the potato a little. You can add a little extra oil if it starts to stick.

Once the peppers have softened, remove the pan from the heat to serve, tearing over the basil leaves if you are using them.

2 tbsp olive oil,
    plus extra if needed
1 red onion,
    roughly chopped
2 garlic cloves,
    roughly chopped
4 potatoes, cut into
    1cm cubes
200g cherry tomatoes,
    roughly chopped
1 red pepper, deseeded
    and roughly chopped
a few basil leaves,
    to serve – optional
salt and pepper

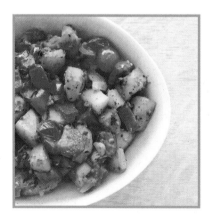

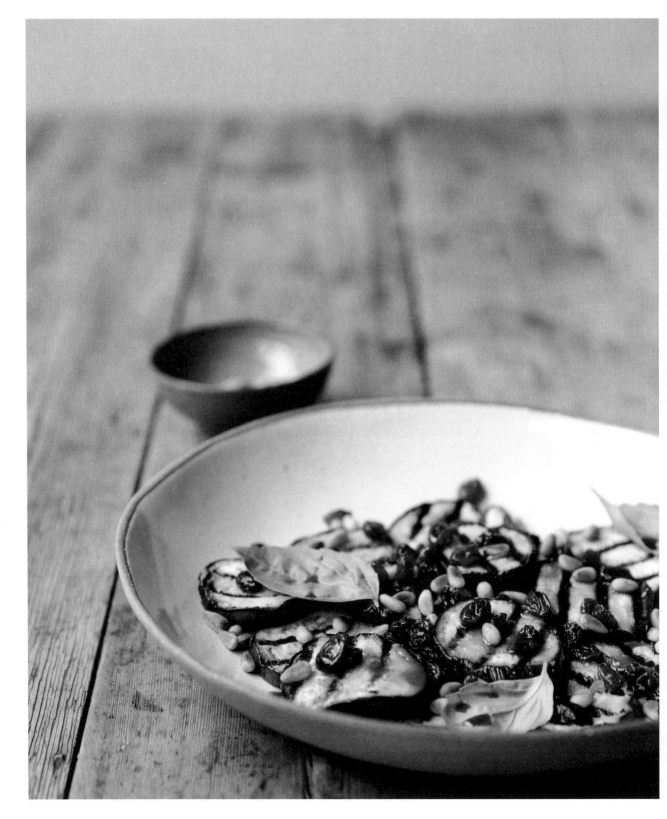

Sweet Grilled Aubergine
with Pine Nuts and Sultanas

I love how versatile aubergine is – you can do so much with it, playing with texture and flavour. This simple dish combines its smoky grilled flavour with a sweet syrup sauce, with pine nuts and sultanas thrown in for added substance. When I first made this, I was so happy with it, but decided to throw in some torn-up basil at the end for good measure and it totally transformed the dish, adding a whole new flavour to the mix.

Slice the aubergine into 1cm thick circles and place them in a mixing bowl. Add a pinch of salt and 1 tablespoon of the olive oil and use your hands to coat the aubergine evenly.

Preheat the grill. Place the aubergine slices under the grill for 5–7 minutes, then turn over and grill for a further 5 minutes until they are soft. (Alternatively, griddle the slices over a high heat for 1–2 minutes on each side.)

While the aubergine cooks, pour the apple cider vinegar into a small pan with the honey over a low heat. Add the sultanas and simmer gently for 5 minutes or until the mixture reduces slightly. Then remove it from the heat and allow to cool and thicken a little. Stir in the remaining 2 tablespoons of olive oil as it cools.

In a small frying pan, lightly toast the pine nuts and then place to one side.

Place the aubergine in a serving dish, then pour over the syrup, sprinkling with pine nuts. Add the basil leaves and mix through the dish to serve.

1 aubergine
3 tbsp olive oil
60ml apple
**   cider vinegar**
2 tsp honey
45g sultanas
20g pine nuts
10g basil leaves
salt

Creamed Spinach

I absolutely love spinach. I find it goes with almost everything and it is so versatile that you can mix it with different spices to make such delicious dishes. This recipe has an Indian influence, inspired by takeaways that I used to enjoy at home with my family and, of course, by the amazing food I had when I was in India during my teacher training.

 This is a great accompaniment to curry dishes, or even just to spice up a rice- or quinoa-veggie combo. If you are short on some of the spices it still works, so don't worry, and feel free to adapt to your own tastes. It is incredibly fragrant and puts a whole new spin on a side of spinach.

1 tsp cumin seeds
1 tsp coriander seeds
2 tbsp olive oil
2 garlic cloves, crushed
½ large or 1 small onion, finely chopped
½ fresh red chilli, deseeded and finely chopped
½ tsp ground turmeric
1cm piece of fresh ginger, peeled and finely chopped
30ml almond milk
150g spinach
½ tsp garam masala – optional

Use the back of a knife to gently crush the cumin and coriander seeds. Heat the oil over a medium heat and add the garlic, onion, crushed cumin and coriander seeds, chilli, turmeric and ginger.

As the onion begins to soften, add the almond milk and the spinach.

If you want to use garam masala to add an extra bit of flavour to the dish, you can do this now, too.

If the spinach begins to dry out as it cooks, add a little extra almond milk or a dash of hot water.

Once the spinach is wilted, it is ready to serve.

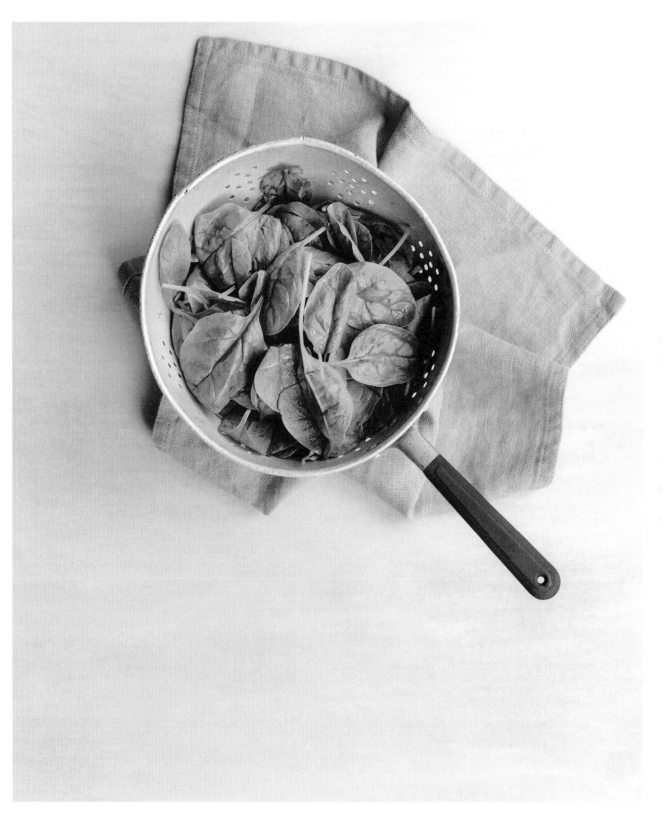

Grilled Avocado with Vine Tomatoes

This couldn't be much simpler, but it makes a delicious side or addition to a lighter salad. Warm avocado sounds strange to some people, but I would urge you to give it a try – I am a big fan.

1 avocado, halved and pitted
14 vine tomatoes, still attached to the vine
1 tsp olive oil
a squeeze of lemon juice
salt and pepper

Preheat the grill. Place the two halves of avocado and the tomatoes under the grill, drizzling with the oil and lemon juice.

Cook for 10 minutes or until the tomato skins begin to split.

Scoop the avocados from their skins – they should come away easily – and serve with the tomatoes.

Season with salt and pepper to serve.

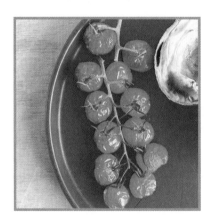

Sesame Roasted Broccoli

This dish is something we eat all the time at home. It was inspired by my best friend, who would probably eat it every day if I didn't insist on him testing my new recipes instead. We like to make it really spicy, so often add extra chilli flakes, but if you don't like spice, you can deseed or leave the fresh chilli out altogether.

Preheat the oven to 180°C/350°F/Gas Mark 4.

Cut the florets off the head of broccoli, then slice them thinly. Slice the broccoli stalk into thin pieces, too – it has lots of flavour. The thinner the pieces, the more crispy they go.

Place the broccoli in a roasting tin with the salt and pepper, and add 30ml of the sesame oil. Mix well to coat the broccoli in the oil. Roast for 10 minutes.

Add the chilli and garlic to the tin, mixing well, and place back in the oven for another 10 minutes.

Finally, add the almonds and the remaining oil, giving everything a stir, before roasting for a further 10 minutes. The broccoli should be crispy around the edges but not burnt.

1 broccoli head
40ml sesame oil
1 fresh red chilli, deseeded if you like, finely chopped
2 garlic cloves, finely chopped
2 tbsp flaked almonds
salt and pepper

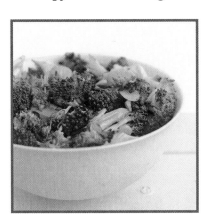

Caramelized Onion and Sweet Potato Cakes

These cakes are a wonderful way to enjoy sweet potato and all of its goodness. They are so full of flavour and are fairly easy to make. The trick is to caramelize the onion well, to bring out the sweetness, as explained in the method below.

600g sweet potatoes, peeled and cut into small chunks
1 red onion, finely sliced
1 tsp coconut oil
1 tsp paprika
½ tsp chilli powder
1 tsp ground cinnamon
olive oil, for frying

Cook the sweet potatoes in a steamer for 20 minutes or until soft. You should be able to mash them easily with a fork.

While the sweet potato steams, place the onion in a saucepan with the coconut oil and mix around so it becomes lightly coated. Leave the onion to caramelize over a low heat for 15–20 minutes. The trick is to stir just enough to stop it from burning, but not too often, as it will interfere with the browning process, which gives that delicious caramel sweetness.

Once the potatoes are soft, transfer them to a mixing bowl and add the paprika, chilli powder and cinnamon. Mash lightly so that they become soft but not totally smooth, then stir in the caramelized onion.

Turn up the heat, add a little olive oil to the pan and take a small ball of the mash in your hands – I usually make about 12 cakes from this mix. If the mash seems really sticky, wash your hands and dry them slightly so that they are still a little damp. Roll the mash in your hands and shape it into a ball, then squash it a little into a roughly 6cm circle. Place it in the pan and repeat with the remaining mix.

Keep an eye on the cakes in the pan, making sure they don't burn. When they have browned on one side, 4 minutes, use a spatula to flip them over and cook for another 4 minutes on the other side. They should be easy to turn. Remove from the heat and serve.

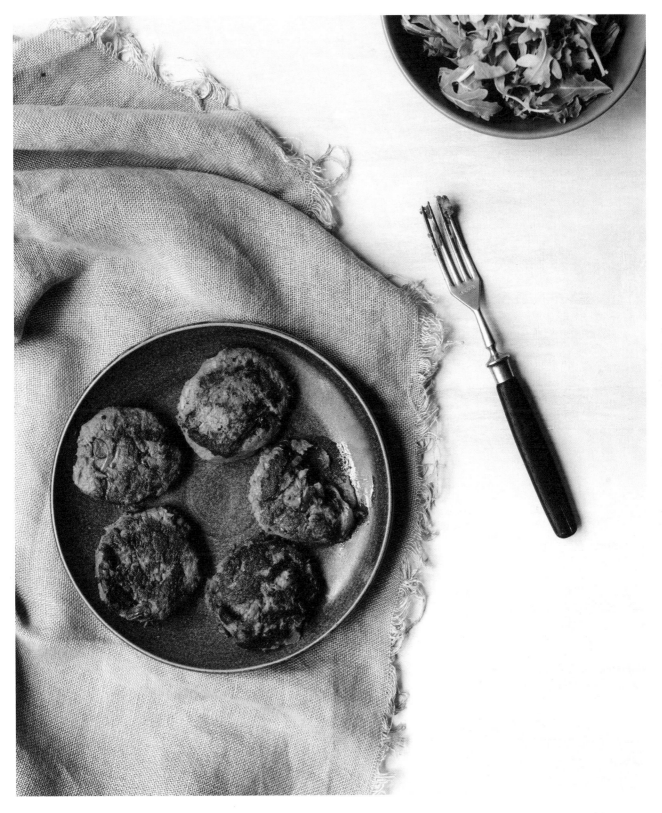

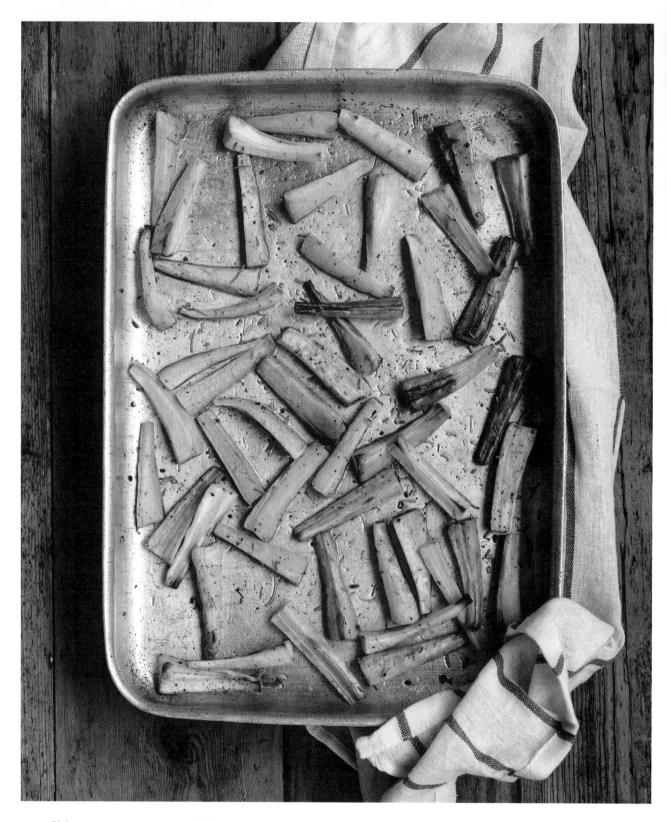

Rosemary Roasted Parsnips

This recipe is a great side dish to add a little comfort to a lighter meal. I often make these to accompany salads, or to enjoy with hummus or other dips. They take just 2 minutes of preparation and minimal attention during cooking but they will fill the kitchen with a delicious smell, making them even more irresistible.

Preheat the oven to 200°C/400°F/Gas Mark 6.

Slice the tips off the parsnips and then cut them in half to separate the thinner and thicker parts. Slice the halves lengthways – making about 3 parts with the lower half and 4–6 with the top.

Place the parsnip slices on a large baking tray and cover with the olive oil and a generous amount of salt and pepper. Spread them out evenly.

Roast the parsnips for 15 minutes, then remove from the oven and add the rosemary. Put them back in the oven for another 15 minutes or until soft, turning a few times so that they cook evenly and don't burn, although I like letting some of them go a little brown and crispy.

Remove from the oven and serve.

500g parsnips
3 tbsp olive oil
2 tsp dried rosemary
salt and pepper

Serves 4 as
a starter, or
2 as a main

Stuffed Mushrooms with Polenta

Cooking with polenta is relatively new to me – in fact, it never really appealed, as it was so unfamiliar. Now I have started using it more, I have actually come to really like it and it is perfect for stuffing mushrooms or other vegetables as it takes on their flavour so well.

100g polenta
1 tsp brown rice
    miso paste
1 red onion, diced
2 garlic cloves, crushed
a little olive oil
1 tsp chilli flakes
4 tsp tahini
4 large mushrooms
    (portobello
    or similar)

Preheat the oven to 180°C/350°F/Gas Mark 4.

Place the polenta, 400ml water and the miso in a saucepan and place over a medium heat, stirring constantly. Once the polenta starts to bubble, after 4 minutes, turn the heat down to the lowest flame and stir every 10 minutes for 35 minutes.

Soften the onion and the garlic in a splash of olive oil. Stir occasionally to prevent them from burning. Once they begin to caramelize, add them to the polenta mix with the chilli flakes. Stir to combine and continue cooking.

Once the polenta is cooked, stir in the tahini.

Preheat the grill, remove the stalks from the mushrooms and then spoon in the polenta mix. Place under the grill for 15 minutes or until the mushrooms are cooked through and the polenta has crisped on the top.

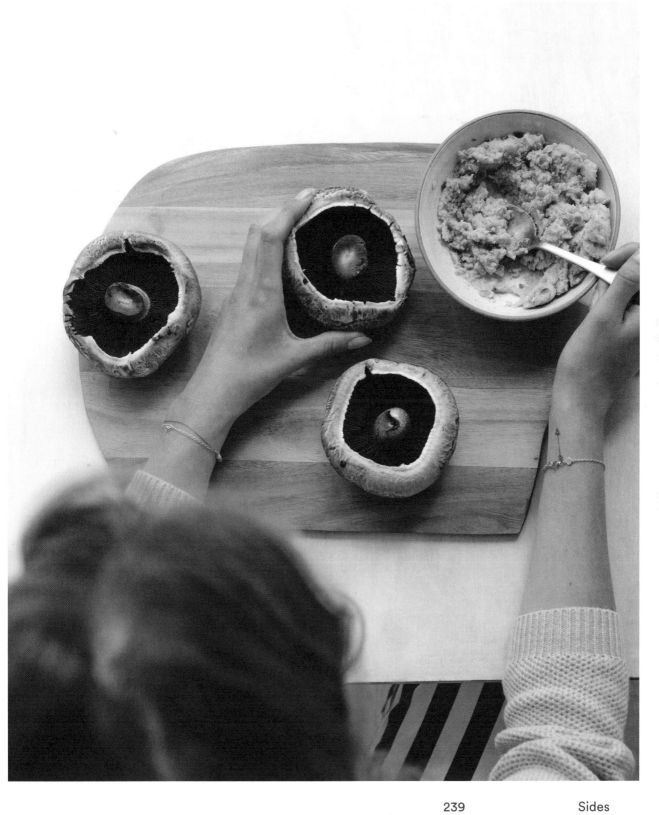

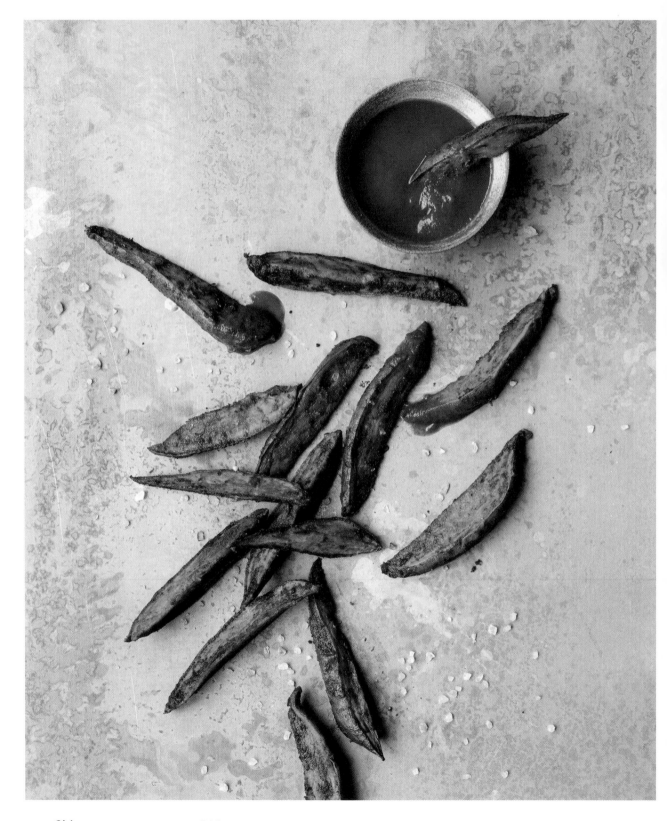

Sweet Potato Wedges with Smoky Ketchup

Sweet potato makes the best wedges because they caramelize slightly, which gives a wonderful sweetness. They crisp on the outside and go totally soft and gooey on the inside. Paired with this smoky ketchup, they are the perfect side, snack or accompaniment to just about anything.

Preheat the oven to 180°C/350°F/Gas Mark 4.

Cut the potatoes into big wedges – I tend to make about eight from a medium sweet potato – then place them on a baking tray. You can peel them if you prefer, but I like to keep the skins on.

In a small pan, melt the coconut oil and mix in the paprika and cinnamon. Pour the mixture over the wedges, seasoning with salt and pepper and using your hands to evenly coat each piece.

Roast for 40 minutes or until soft but retaining enough structure that they can be picked up (keeping the skins on will help).

In the meantime, you can make the ketchup. Place all the ingredients in a small pan over a low heat and add 50ml water, then stir well. Cook until it reduces and thickens to a ketchup consistency. You can serve it warm or cold, whatever you prefer.

Once the wedges are done, remove them from the oven, sprinkle with some salt, and serve immediately.

For the wedges
2 sweet potatoes, unpeeled
2 tbsp coconut oil
2 tsp paprika
1 tsp ground cinnamon
salt and pepper

For the ketchup
2 tbsp tomato purée
1 tsp tamari
3 tsp maple syrup
½ tsp paprika
a pinch of salt

Quinoa Tabbouleh

When I began experimenting with food, my go-to meal was always quinoa with lots of vegetables. I used to roast big batches once or twice a week and then go back to them again and again for packed lunches and easy dinners. Some days, for something a little fresher, I would cut up raw tomatoes, cucumber or whatever else was in the fridge and mix them in with a squeeze of lemon.

Now that I'm more confident combining flavours and experimenting with different ingredients, I don't visit this recipe as much, but I've shared it as I want people to see how easy this sort of cooking can be. I've played around with it a bit over time, and love adding fresh herbs and spices. I've never been that enthusiastic about parsley, but it really brings out the other flavours in this dish, making it a great addition.

150g quinoa
225g tomatoes,
    finely chopped
4 spring onions,
    finely chopped
1 tsp finely chopped
    parsley leaves
1 tsp finely chopped
    mint leaves
salt and pepper

For the dressing
juice of 1 lemon
3 tbsp olive oil
¼ tsp ground cinnamon
¼ tsp grated nutmeg
¼ tsp ground coriander

Place the quinoa in a pan with a pinch of salt, and fill with water to one thumb's width higher than the quinoa. Bring to the boil and simmer for 10 minutes, then turn off the heat and place a lid over the pan. Leave for 10 minutes, then fluff with a fork. If there is any excess water, drain it and set aside to cool.

Place the tomatoes and spring onions in a mixing bowl, along with any tomato juice that squeezes out. Then mix in the quinoa and herbs once it has cooled.

To make the dressing, put all the dressing ingredients in a small bowl and stir well.

Pour the dressing into the mixing bowl and stir everything through thoroughly, seasoning before serving.

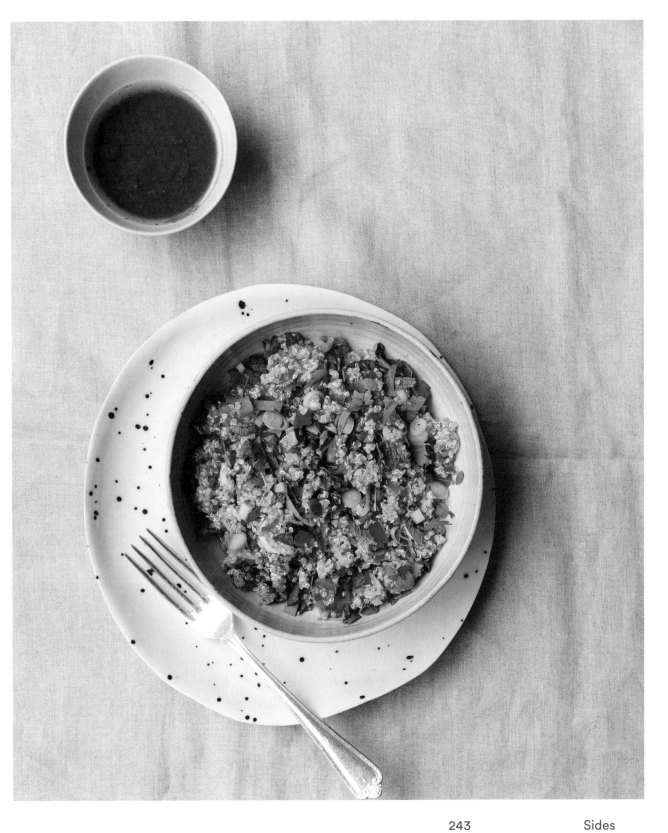

Sides

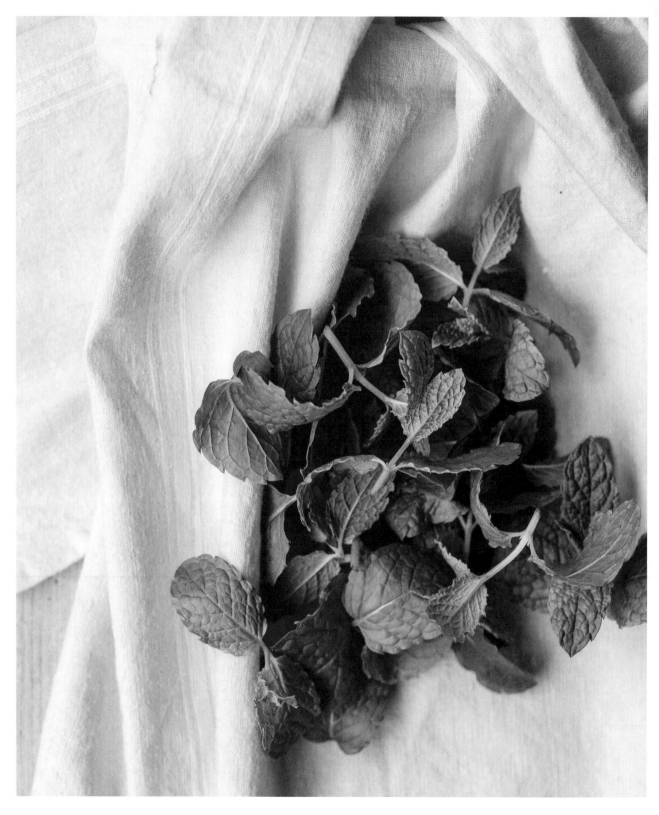

Pea and Mint Pesto

This is one of my absolute favourite things to keep in the fridge. It goes with pretty much everything and I love to spoon it onto salads, cook it with beans or mix it into a bowl of quinoa or pasta.

Pesto pasta was a childhood favourite, but most pre-bought jars contain cheese or other ingredients that I don't eat any more. Luckily, making your own is wonderfully simple and you have the freedom to make it completely to your own taste. Sometimes I add a little extra lemon, or make it more minty depending on what I fancy.

Boil some salted water and then add the peas, cover and simmer for 3 minutes. Drain and run them under cold water to cool down before moving on to the next step.

Add the peas to a food processor with all the other ingredients. Blend well until you have your desired consistency. I like to make it pretty smooth, but it also works really well if you prefer it a little chunky.

Store in a sealed container in the fridge for up to 1 week.

250g frozen peas
leaves from
    7 mint stalks
juice of 1 lemon
75g almonds
100ml olive oil
salt and pepper

Carrot and Tarragon Purée

This is a really simple side dish, perfect for adding to Buddha-style bowls or for using as a dip. The fresh tarragon gives it an aromatic flavour, complementing the sweetness of the carrots and keeping it feeling light and fresh.

500g carrots, cut
into 1cm pieces
½ tsp chopped
tarragon leaves
2 tsp tahini
juice of ½ lemon
salt and pepper

Place the carrots in a steamer and cook over a medium–high heat for 25 minutes or until completely soft.

Rinse the carrots under a cold tap to cool, then transfer them to a food processor. Add the remaining ingredients and blend until smooth.

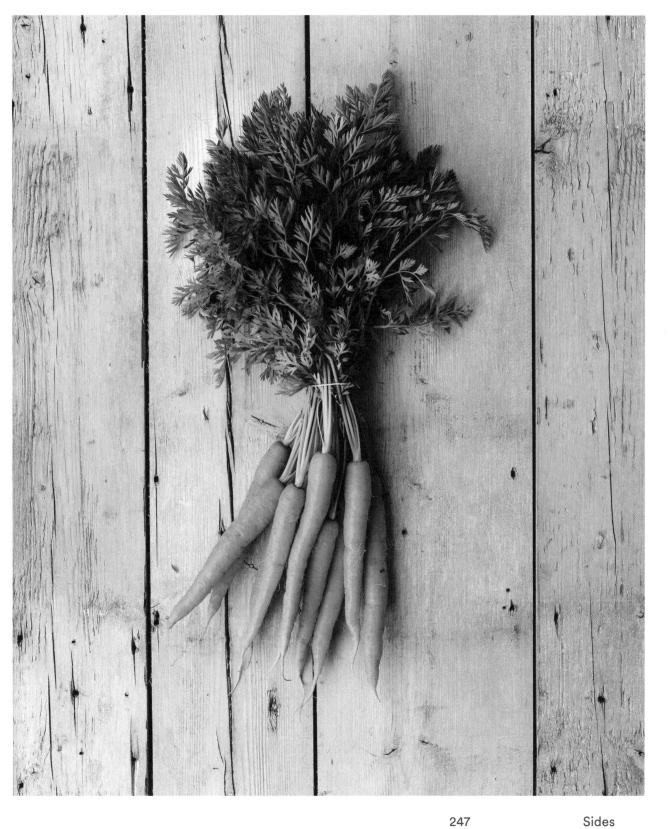

Sides

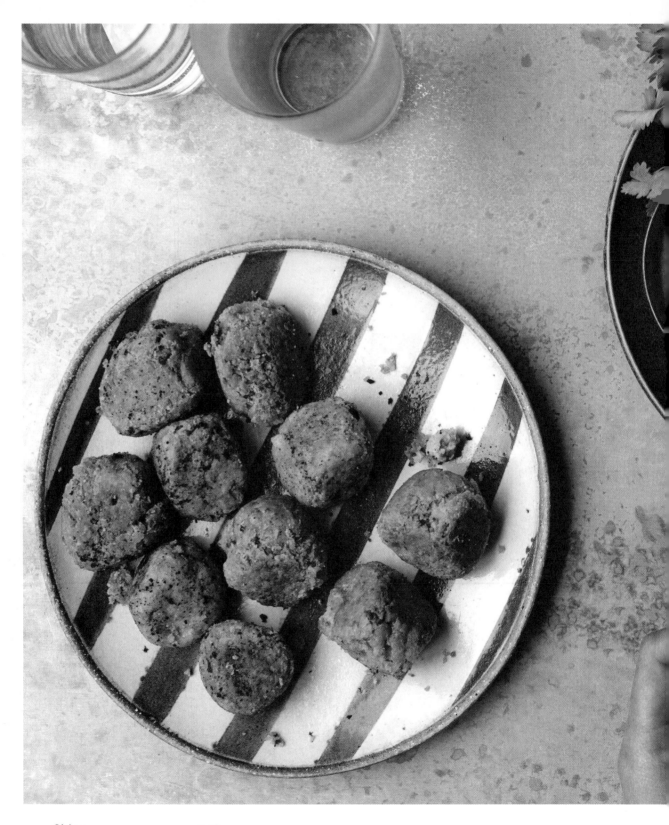

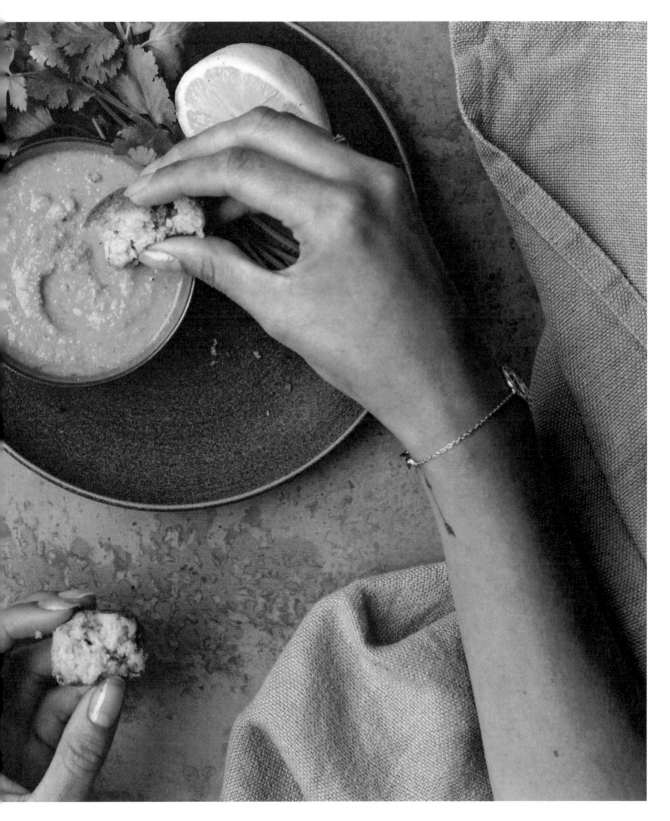

Pea Falafel with Spicy Tomato Dipping Sauce

This is a spin on the classic falafel – the same, but greener! I love the sweetness of the peas, and the lemon zest complements the sauce perfectly, to which the cashews add a little thickness. In fact, the sauce makes a great addition to any simple salad.

For the falafel
200g frozen peas
400g tin chickpeas,
    drained and rinsed
2 tbsp gram flour
1 garlic clove
1 tsp ground cumin
1 tbsp tahini
1 tbsp olive oil,
    plus extra for frying
zest of ½ lemon
salt and pepper

For the dipping sauce
½ tsp ground cumin
40g cashews
½ tsp chilli flakes
350g tomatoes, diced
2 garlic cloves, diced

Boil a kettle, pour the water over the peas and then leave for 2 minutes to defrost them. Place in a food processor with the remaining falafel ingredients and blend for 30 seconds so that you have a chunky mixture. Be careful not to leave it too long as you don't want to let it go too smooth.

Using wet hands, take a small ball of the mixture and roll it between your palms, then squash it a little to flatten the edges. Repeat this step for the remaining mixture, then place all the balls on a plate in the fridge for 10 minutes to set – you should have around 12.

In the meantime, make the sauce. In a small pan, gently heat the cumin, cashews and chilli flakes for 1 minute or until the nuts brown. Remove from the heat and leave to one side. Heat the tomatoes and garlic gently in the pan for a few minutes until the tomatoes soften and start to break down.

Remove the tomatoes from the heat and pour into a blender with the cashews in their spices. Blend until smooth. You can choose to let the dipping sauce cool, or place it back in the pan to heat through before serving.

Add a generous amount of olive oil to the pan and carefully fry the falafels – you may need to do so in batches depending on the size of the pan. Cook for a minute or so on each side, or until golden brown, then remove from the heat, draining any excess oil. Serve with the dipping sauce.

05

pick-me-ups for those peckish moments

snacks

Banana Bread

This is one of my earliest blog recipes and it's been a hit time and time again. I'm not a natural baker and this positive feedback came as a welcome surprise. So for anyone who usually shies away from baking, I encourage you to try this banana bread – it doesn't need a food processor and there are no raw eggs involved, so you really can't go wrong. It's meant to be dense, and when you take it out of the oven it might not look totally set but it will firm up after a few minutes. Depending on the ripeness of the bananas you use, you can add a little maple syrup to sweeten it more, but I find it sweet enough as it is. If you can keep it hidden well enough, it lasts for up to a week in a sealed container (although that never seems to happen in my house!).

30g chia seeds
3 overripe bananas
200g Medjool
   dates, pitted
1 tsp maca powder
   – optional
1 tsp ground cinnamon
150g buckwheat flour
200g ground almonds
150ml almond milk

Preheat the oven to 180°C/350°F/Gas Mark 4.

Start by soaking the chia seeds in 60ml water. Stir well and place to one side until a gel forms.

Next, peel the bananas, then take one and slice it lengthways. Save one half for the top, then mash the remaining half with the other two (so 2½ bananas in total) in a large mixing bowl.

Chop the dates roughly (I like to use scissors to do this), then add all the other ingredients, except for the almond milk, to the mixing bowl with 60ml water and mix. Once they have come together, begin to add the almond milk little by little until the mixture is sticky but still solid enough to slightly hold its shape.

Line a loaf tin or small, deep baking tin (16 x 26cm) with baking parchment and pour in the mix. Finally, press the halved banana on the top.

Bake the bread for 45 minutes, then leave to cool for 10 minutes before slicing.

Toffee Popcorn

I love cosy evenings in with friends, snuggled up on the sofa, watching a movie or just catching up, but always with a big bowl of popcorn to pick at. We make this far too often at home, and get through far more of it than we would want to admit, but it has definitely taken a while to master the technique. The trouble when using coconut oil is that you risk making the popcorn soggy, but I have finally worked out all the tricks to leave you with a delicious bowlful to share with friends.

Pour the popcorn kernels into a large saucepan, then cover with a lid over a medium heat. Occasionally shake the pan to keep the heat even and prevent any burning. Keep an eye on the corn to make sure that it doesn't start to brown or burn, and adjust the heat accordingly.

Once the popcorn starts jumping (more than the first few), you can remove it from the heat until the popping stops. If lots of the kernels haven't popped, you can heat it again. Then remove the lid and transfer the popcorn to a mixing bowl to cool.

In a small pan, add the remaining ingredients and stir gently over a low heat until the coconut sugar has dissolved. Before it starts to bubble, turn off the heat and leave the sauce to thicken for a minute

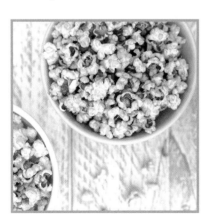

or two. Then pour over the popcorn, stirring well until it is evenly coated. Leave it to set (if you can) for 10 minutes before serving.

150g popcorn kernels
3 tbsp maple syrup
3 tbsp coconut sugar
1½ tsp coconut oil
a large pinch of pink
    Himalayan salt

Hot Chocolate

Everyone loves hot chocolate, right? Well, this one is also good for you! With no added sweetener, the milk, coconut oil and vanilla combine to make a beautifully indulgent but light version of this family favourite.

250ml almond or
  brown rice milk
½ tsp coconut oil
2 tsp raw cacao powder
¼ tsp vanilla powder

Heat the milk gently on the hob, adding the coconut oil and raw cacao and vanilla powders.

Stir well until the milk is hot and the powders have dissolved, but it is not yet boiling.

Pour into a mug to serve.

Serves 1

Turmeric Latte

250ml coconut milk,
  brown rice or
  almond milk
¼ tsp ground turmeric
a pinch of grated nutmeg
  (or ½ tsp honey)
  – optional
cracked black pepper

I know turmeric can be a bit of an acquired taste, so this one may seem a little strange, but I would encourage you not to knock it before you've tried it! I have been totally converted to these and now absolutely love them mid-morning or as an afternoon drink instead of a coffee. Adding nutmeg really brings a whole different taste and smell to the drink, but you can opt for honey to sweeten it instead if you prefer.

In a small pan, combine all the ingredients and warm over a low heat. Stir gently until the milk is hot, but not boiling. Transfer the golden turmeric milk to a mug to serve.

Matcha Latte

Matcha green tea powder always looked pretty off-putting, until I discovered how good it can taste in a drink. By combining the powder with brown rice milk for sweetness and spicing it with cinnamon, you get a delicious latte that gives a wonderful energy boost, making it a great mid-morning or afternoon pick-me-up. It is the perfect replacement for coffee if you are trying to cut down and the sweetness will help satisfy that sugar craving, too.

Add the matcha powder and 1 teaspoon boiling water to a mug and stir well to form a paste.

In a small saucepan, gently heat the milk. Allow it to reach the point where it is simmering gently, then remove it from the heat and stir in ½ teaspoon cinnamon. I like to use a small electric frother to froth the milk, but there is no need to if you don't have one.

Pour the milk into your mug and whisk to fully incorporate. Top with the remaining cinnamon.

1 tsp matcha green tea powder
250ml brown rice milk or almond milk (you may like to sweeten with ½–1 tsp honey if you use almond milk)
½–1 tsp ground cinnamon

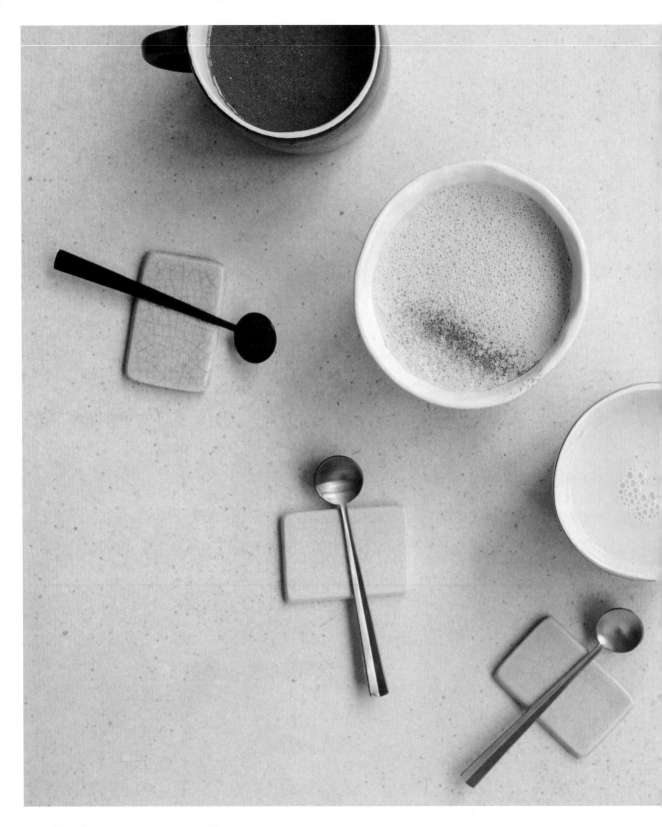

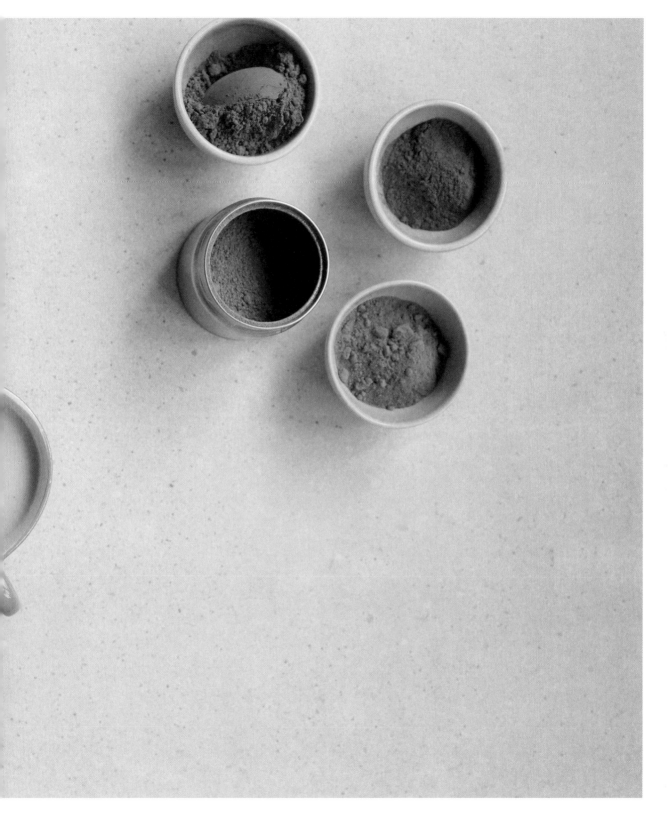

Baked Banana with Chocolate Sauce

I'm not really a dessert person, but this dish is so simple that it makes a perfect treat to enjoy after dinner when you fancy something sweet with minimal effort. The chocolate sauce is completely delicious – you'll probably struggle not to just eat it with a spoon!

4 bananas
1 lemon, quartered
2 tsp vanilla powder
30g flaked almonds

For the chocolate sauce
5 Medjool dates, pitted
250ml almond milk
2 tbsp raw
    cacao powder
½ tsp ground
    cardamom or 1
    cardamom pod

Preheat the oven to 180°C/350°F/Gas Mark 4.

Peel the bananas and place each one in a piece of foil. Squeeze a quarter of a lemon on each and sprinkle with vanilla. Wrap them up in their foil packets and cook in the oven for 10 minutes.

While the bananas cook, make the chocolate sauce. Place the dates in a blender with the almond milk and whizz until smooth. Pour into a saucepan over a low heat and stir in the raw cacao powder and cardamom. Let it warm up, but not bubble or burn. Keep stirring while it heats through to remove any lumps of cacao. Remove the cardamom pod, if using.

In a small dry pan, toast the flaked almonds until they begin to turn golden brown, then remove from the heat and place to one side.

Remove the bananas from the oven and place them in bowls or on small plates. Drizzle over the chocolate sauce and sprinkle with the almonds to serve.

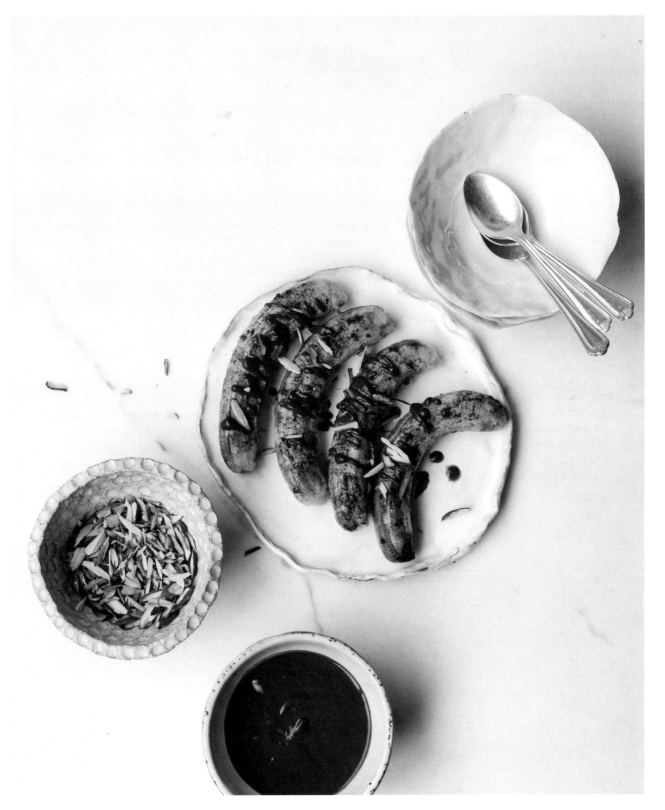

Chocolate Orange Energy Balls

Energy balls are such a fantastic thing to keep in the fridge or freezer, ready for a sugar craving or to give you a little energy boost during the day. These are inspired by the winning flavour combination of chocolate and orange, giving them a zesty and decadent taste.

200g almonds
200g Medjool dates, pitted (I like to have a few extra dates to hand in case the mixture isn't quite sticky enough, as it can vary a little each batch)
zest and juice of 1 orange
2 tbsp raw cacao powder
2 tbsp maple syrup

Blend the almonds in a food processor to break them into smaller pieces. Add the dates, whizzing for a minute or so.

Add all the orange zest and 1 tablespoon of the juice to the food processor, along with the raw cacao and the maple syrup, before mixing until evenly distributed.

Try a little of the mixture, adding extra orange juice if needed.

Use your hands to roll the mixture in your palms (wetting your hands slightly if necessary) until you have about 16 even-sized balls. Place them in the fridge or freezer to set and store. They will keep for 1 week in the fridge and for 2 weeks in the freezer.

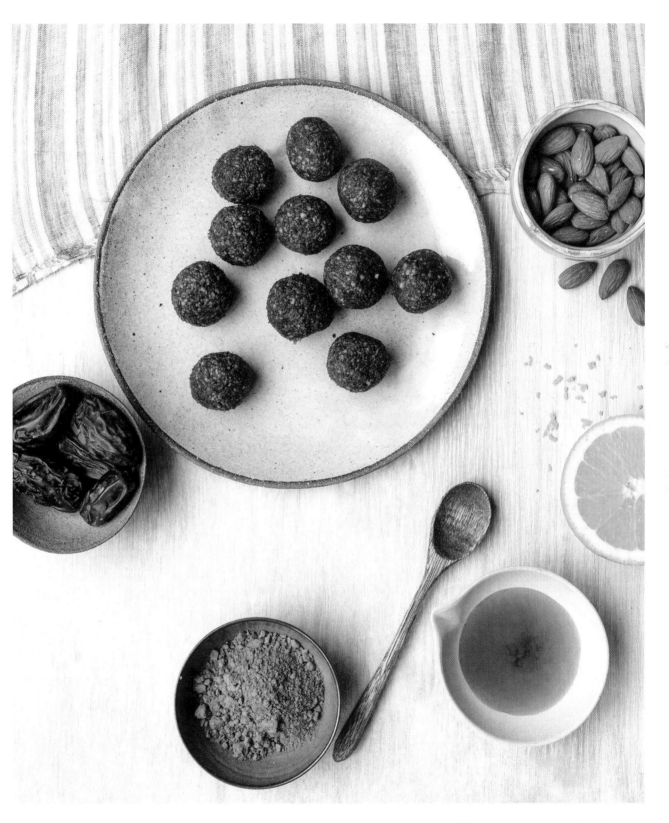

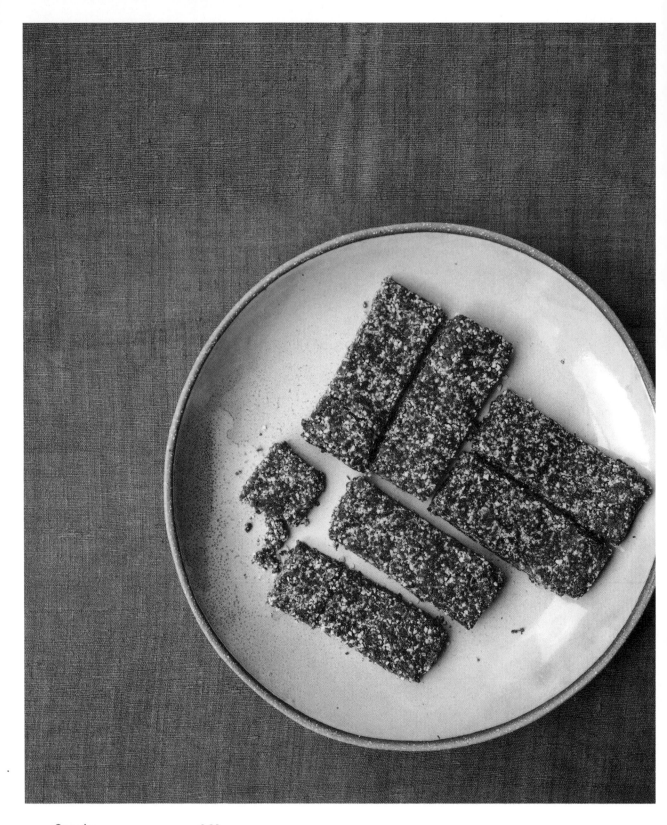

Hemp Protein Bars

Makes 12
small bars

These bars are a real staple, perfect for an active day to give you a little protein hit. You can buy hemp powder online and it works really well in this recipe, in which the dates and tahini give the perfect amount of sweet and saltiness. The almonds provide extra protein, too, filling you up in between meals and helping your body to recover from workouts or generally busy days.

Whizz the almonds in a food processor until they have broken down into tiny pieces, stopping before it forms a flour.

If the dates don't feel soft and sticky, you can soak them in boiling water for a few minutes to help them hold the mixture together. Add the dates to the food processor with the tahini and protein powder, and blend to make a thick and slightly sticky mixture.

While everything is blending, line a shallow 20 × 30cm baking tray with cling film. Empty the mixture onto the tray and use a spatula to pack the mixture tightly to make sure it is well stuck together and not crumbly.

Use a sharp knife to cut the mixture into 12 equal bars. If you have packed the mixture well enough, they should cut easily without falling apart at all. (Alternatively, you can roll them into balls if you prefer.)

Place the bars in the fridge to set for 20 minutes. I like to then wrap them in baking parchment to stop them from sticking together and then I store them in a plastic box in the fridge for up to 1 week.

200g almonds
200g Medjool dates, pitted (it's good to have a few extra in case the mixture is a little bit crumbly)
1 tbsp tahini
60g hemp protein powder

Chocolate Mousse

As children we absolutely loved chocolate mousse. I can't even begin to count the number of times we tried to sneak a second pot and have a competition to see who could savour it the longest because it was so easy to just wolf it down.

This is the quickest dessert. It only takes about 2 minutes to make and requires no blender or food processor – do remember to pop the coconut milk in the fridge the night before, though. You can make the mousse in advance and keep it in the fridge – just allow it to stand for a few minutes before serving and then give it a fluff with a fork if it has solidified. The coconut milk needs to be 100 per cent coconut from a brand such as Biona so that the water separates from the solid. This does happen in some tins that are 60–70 per cent coconut, but often they contain lots of emulsifiers, which I like to avoid. You can add more sweetener and less cacao for a milkier feel, or up the cacao and reduce the maple if you prefer dark chocolate.

400ml tin coconut milk, chilled upright
3 tsp raw cacao powder
1–2 tsp maple syrup, to taste
berries and desiccated coconut, to serve – optional

Open the tin of coconut milk and scoop out the solid part from the top, placing it in a mixing bowl. Discard the liquid part or save it for a smoothie.

Add the raw cacao and maple syrup (I like to start with less and add more if needed).

Use a fork to whisk it all together, then serve. I love to add berries and desiccated coconut to serve, but it's delicious on its own, too.

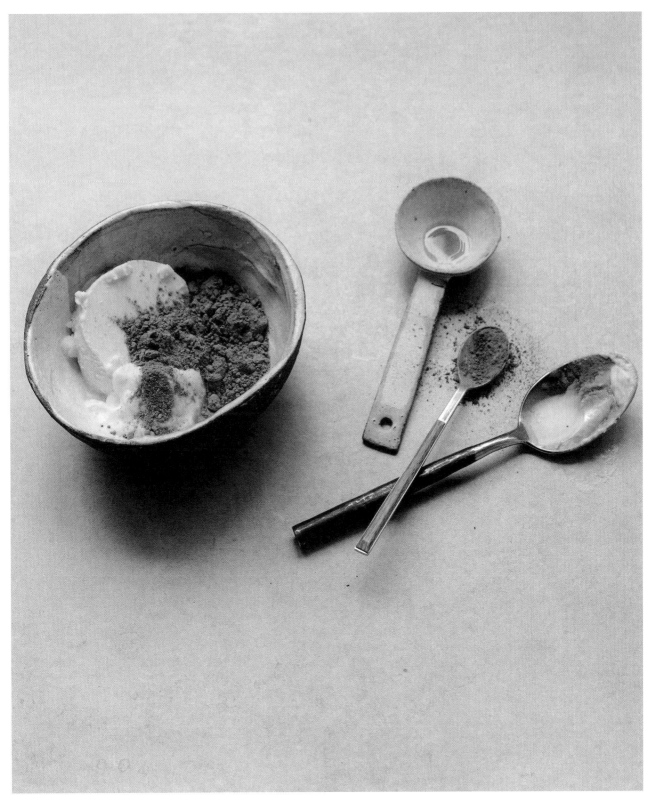

Index

Page references in *italics* indicate photographs.

Acknowledgements

It feels really quite amazing to see this book come together and I couldn't be more grateful to everyone who has supported me in sharing my journey. It is rare that we take the time to sit back and really take stock of the people and loved ones around us, but this process has helped me think about what a wonderful support network I have.

There are a few people who I would like to thank who have really been there for me – not just during the writing of this book but in the process that lead me to writing it, starting with my family. I would like to thank them for their unconditional love and support, and for allowing me to find my own way, while offering guidance and space in perfect measures to help me grow into the person I am today.

To Will, for questioning every step, for being there and for making sure I am always the best, most authentic version of myself. I couldn't have done any of this without you. Thank you for everything and for letting me use some of your photography, too!

Ella and Olivia – you inspired me to embark on this process and I will always be so thankful to have you both in my life and for giving me the kick I needed to explore what it was I really believed in and wanted to share. Lotte, you are such a special friend and your integrity is a real inspiration. And to all my other friends who have supported and cared for me along the way – each of you mean the world to me. Thank you for being there.

To my agent, Rachel, who believed in this even before there was a book and who helped me to grow what I have learned into something worth sharing. To the wonderful team who created such beautiful images – Philippa, Uyen, Lydia, Maria and Cynthia, I had such fun working with you all. To my editor, Carolyn, for her guidance through the whole process and for investing in me and this book, and Lucy – this design is so beautiful. Thank you all for sharing my vision and helping to bring it to life. To Zoe, Polly, Orlando, George, Helena, Jan and everyone else at HarperCollins for all the hard work you all put in along the way. I am truly grateful to each of you.

And finally, to each and every reader of my blog, who have helped turn a hobby into a living, and to my yoga teachers and students for inspiring me every single day. I love hearing from and about you all and feel so lucky to be able to learn and share with you as we discover new things and grow a little each day. I hope I can continue to share this journey with you all for a long time to come.

Conversion Charts

Dry weights

METRIC	IMPERIAL	METRIC	IMPERIAL
5g	¼oz	500g	1lb 2oz
8/10g	⅓oz	550g	1lb 3oz
15g	½oz	600g	1lb 5oz
20g	¾oz	625g	1lb 6oz
25g	1oz	650g	1lb 7oz
30/35g	1¼oz	675g	1½lb
40g	1½oz	700g	1lb 9oz
50g	2oz	750g	1lb 10oz
60/70g	2½oz	800g	1¾lb
75/85/90g	3oz	850g	1lb 14oz
100g	3½oz	900g	2lb
110/120g	4oz	950g	2lb 2oz
125/130g	4½oz	1kg	2lb 3oz
135/140/150g	5oz	1.1kg	2lb 6oz
170/175g	6oz	1.25kg	2¾lb
200g	7oz	1.3/1.4kg	3lb
225g	8oz	1.5kg	3lb 5oz
250g	9oz	1.75/1.8kg	4lb
265g	9½oz	2kg	4lb 4oz
275g	10oz	2.25kg	5lb
300g	11oz	2.5kg	5½lb
325g	11½oz	3kg	6½lb
350g	12oz	3.5kg	7¾lb
375g	13oz	4kg	8¾lb
400g	14oz	4.5kg	9¾lb
425g	15oz	6.8kg	15lb
450g	1lb	9kg	20lb
475g	1lb 1oz		

Liquid Measures

568ml = 1 UK pint (20fl oz) | 16fl oz = 1 US pint

METRIC	IMPERIAL	CUPS	METRIC	IMPERIAL	CUPS
15ml	½fl oz	1 tbsp (level)	425ml	15fl oz	
20ml	¾fl oz		450ml	16fl oz	2 cups
25ml	1fl oz	⅛ cup	500ml	18fl oz	2¼ cups
30ml	1¼fl oz		550ml	19fl oz	
50ml	2fl oz	¼ cup	600ml	1 pint	2½ cups
60ml	2½fl oz		700ml	1¼ pints	
75ml	3fl oz		750ml	1⅓pints	
100ml	3½fl oz	⅜ cup	800ml	1 pint 9fl oz	
110/120ml	4fl oz	½ cup	850ml	1½ pints	
125ml	4½fl oz		900ml	1 pint 12fl oz	3¾ cups
150ml	5fl oz	⅔ cup	1 litre	1¾ pints	1 US quart (4 cups)
175ml	6fl oz	¾ cup	1.2 litres	2 pints	1¼ US quarts
200/215ml	7fl oz		1.25 litres	2¼ pints	
225ml	8fl oz	1 cup	1.5 litres	2½ pints	3 US pints
250ml	9fl oz		1.75/1.8 litres	3 pints	
275ml	9½fl oz		2 litres	3½ pints	2 US quarts
300ml	½ pint	1¼ cups	2.2 litres	3¾ pints	
350ml	12fl oz	1½ cups	2.5 litres	4⅓ pints	
375ml	13fl oz		3 litres	5 pints	
400ml	14fl oz		3.5 litres	6 pints	

Oven temperatures

All recipes are based on fan-assisted oven temperatures. If you are using a conventional oven, raise the temperature 20°C higher than stated in recipes.

°C	°F	GAS MARK	DESCRIPTION
110	225	¼	cool
130	250	½	cool
140	275	1	very low
150	300	2	very low
160/170	325	3	low to moderate
180	350	4	moderate
190	375	5	moderately hot
200	400	6	hot
220	425	7	hot
230	450	8	hot
240	475	9	very hot

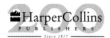

Thorsons
An imprint of HarperCollins*Publishers*
1 London Bridge Street
London SE1 9GF

www.harpercollins.co.uk

First published by Thorsons 2017

10 9 8 7 6 5 4 3 2 1

Text © Annie Clarke 2017
Photography © Philippa Langley 2017
Instagram photography courtesy of the author and Will Sebastian

Annie Clarke asserts the moral right to be identified as the author of this work

Food styling Frankie Unsworth
Prop styling: Linda Berlin
Hair and make-up: Frances Done
Clothes styling: Annie Swain

A catalogue record of this book is available from the British Library

ISBN 978-0-00-819110-8

Printed and bound in China

MIX
Paper from
responsible sources
FSC FSC™ C007454
www.fsc.org

FSC™ is a non-profit international organisation established to promote the
responsible management of the world's forests. Products carrying the FSC
label are independently certified to assure consumers that they come from
forests that are managed to meet the social, economic and ecological needs
of present and future generations, and other controlled sources.

Find out more about HarperCollins and the environment at
www.harpercollins.co.uk/green